WOMEN WHO BOSSUP

WOMEN WHO
BossUp

Secrets of Success From
Women Who Have Leveled Up
in Life, Health and Business

PRESENTED BY

Women With Vision International

First Printing, 2020

Book Interior Design by VMC Art & Design

ISBN 978-0-9992060-7-2
Library of Congress Control Number: 2020916066

Delucslife Media
Cerritos, CA 90703

www.delucslife.com

Printed in China

TABLE OF CONTENTS

INTRODUCTION:

Girl Talk
with Tam Luc

═══════════════════════════

THE ENTIRE YEAR of 2019, we were optimistic. The thinking was, man, 2020 is almost here and it's going to be great.

Actually, for much of the last 10 years, I felt that 2020 meant something. It was going to be a new beginning, where we could see clearly something great. I believe a lot of people felt that way. But the reality has been far from what we expected.

January 26, 2020, Kobe Bryant dies in a helicopter crash along with his daughter and seven other passengers. Nobody saw that coming. Kobe Bryant was loved by people globally, so we all saw the news and felt its impact. Kobe represented excellence. Not just black excellence, but excellence in mind and game. I don't know many people who have worked as hard as he did on his craft. He represented winning. He wasn't a perfect human, but watching him transition to dedicated husband, completely present father, and capable businessman was inspiring. And I don't even think I realized how much he inspired me until he passed away.

Every community around the world was affected by the news. And so, 2020 started off with global attention on someone who had touched us all. Then... COVID-19, the disease caused by a novel coronavirus that originated in Wuhan, China, in late 2019, became a global pandemic. Never in my lifetime has every individual been so impacted by an infectious disease. Other diseases always seemed to be someone else's problem. We weren't unaware of pandemics but the last one in the US was about a hundred years ago. The flu pandemic of 1918, known as the Spanish Flu, a strain that originated from birds, was long forgotten." More recent infectious diseases such as HIV, SARS, and others, had not affected daily life on such a massive scale in our country. And now we find ourselves confined in quarantine, hoarding toilet paper, and ordering $100 paper masks. We've experienced an incredible disruption in all aspects of our lives. Our family and business plans, including all travel, were canceled instantly. And I witnessed genuine fear on people's faces. Protests erupted because people did not believe they needed to change their lifestyle. No masks, no quarantines, you can't make me.

And then the Black Lives Matter movement experienced a great resurgence. Once again, another black man was killed at the hands of the police. The killing of George Floyd set off a global cry that could not be unheard. Mr. Floyd was not a perfect human, but he was a man who didn't need to die. We all saw the tape. This was the tipping point. No one, globally, could unsee the horrific 8 minutes and 46 seconds. Civil unrest erupted in the streets. Protests from the anger of constant killing. Most of these, peaceful demonstrations and marches that still continue day after day. The outpouring ignited protests in Australia, New Zealand, UK, Canada, Germany, Denmark, and Japan. So, the first six months of 2020 was interesting.

Six months. Yes, what we do is affecting each other. Now, what can we do to support global community healing? To find out, I turned to women leaders, whom I have a special affinity with and belief in, for stories of triumph, confidence, and faith.

In the beginning of the pandemic, there was a woman protesting the stay-at-home order. She was not happy and perceived that the real threat was her inability to go to work. She was frantic. She was upset. She was yelling at a newscaster. "I need to go to work to feed my family," she yelled. My first thought was, "Wow, is she crazy? People are dying. Get ahold of yourself." Then I realized. That is fear. She was genuinely scared and unable to see any way to support herself and her family other than going to work in a pandemic. She was stuck.

I remember being stuck in 2008 during the economic crisis in the US. It took me a while to get it together. What I needed—what the woman protesting the stay-at-home order needed—was a "girl talk." *Come on, now. You can do this. Come on, girl. You got it in you to do this.* And that is what this book is. I know there are women out there who need some "girl talk" to believe in themselves again. To BossUp no matter what the situation—not just pandemics, but abuse and divorce and homelessness and their own stinking thinking.

The term BossUp is quite intuitive and can be interpreted but this American slang means **"To begin to act or approach something with resolve, determination, and all of one's effort. If I really wanted that promotion, I knew I was going to have to boss up. You'll need to start bossing up if you want to get your idea off the ground."** BossUp is meant to not only honor women, but also to inspire and empower all women, no matter what their situation.

You know you can do it because other women have done the same.

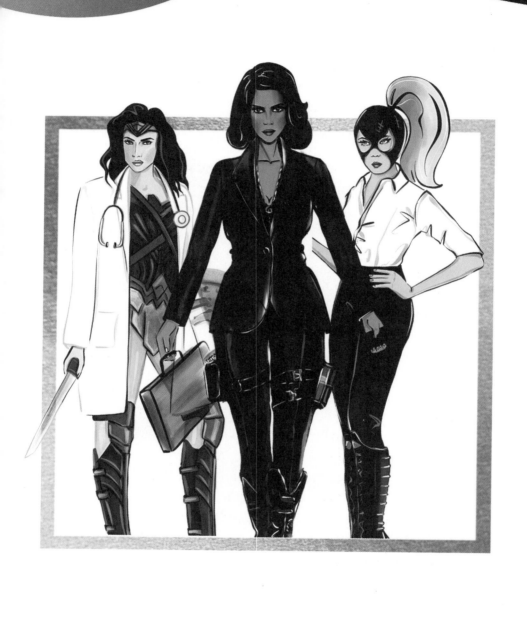

SECTION 1:
Women Who BossUp

"Their are no
failures only
lessons."

—TAM LUC

CHAPTER 1:

What does it mean?
with Tam Luc

HEY, THERE SUPERWOMEN. I am excited about our new season and the many things that I've learned over the past year and a half since starting the podcast. I can't even believe it's been that long. Women With Vision is truly a passion but many want to know *Why did I start Women With Vision?*

Women with Vision is all about uplifting and empowering women to be who they want to be, do whatever they want to do and know that they can—no matter what the situation is. It doesn't matter if they're married or single or have been through some ups and downs. We are here to share our similar experiences and empower each other. "Women with Vision" is a response to some of the things that I learned along my journey. Before answering, I'm going to go a little further back and take you on a little walk through my life. I will share where I've been, where I'm planning to go—and I want you to go with me.

I hope you guys are enjoying yourself being on this ride with me—so here goes. I'm originally from Cincinnati, Ohio. I was born in Pittsburgh, Pennsylvania and my parents moved from Pittsburgh to Cleveland, Ohio early in their marriage. I lived there for a very short time until my mom got divorced from my biological dad and then moved down to Cincinnati. I'm the oldest of three children. If you haven't noticed, I'm a bit bossy, pretty opinionated, and very responsible—I have this older sibling thing going. I have always been a mama hen or mother hen to most of my friends and that comes from watching my mother as well as having a lot of responsibility when I was young.

My mom came from a really small town in Northern Ohio and my father came from Pittsburgh. My dad was a very good looking dude—think about the *Debarges*. Every time I see the singing group *The Debarges* I see my dad—he was good looking. My mom was a beautiful woman. Based on her account, the main reason for the attraction to him was because he's a pretty man. He ended up being a really terrible abusive person with a lot of issues.

At the time, it was me and my sister. A situation happened when I was young where I saw my mom being physically abused by my dad. I watched that happen—it was terrible and I never forgot it. I believe that situation—was why she decided to leave him. She did not want to raise her daughters to see that kind of abuse and believe that was normal. She did not want to be in that kind of life, she didn't think she deserved that, and neither did she want her children to see that. When she decided and finally got enough courage to leave him, she found out she was pregnant with my brother so—here she is... with three little kids. I was four, my sister was two, and my brother was a newborn. So she ran away and left him.

He did not take it well so she had to run for her life with three toddlers in tow. I can't even imagine how difficult that had to be. A young woman having to move from Cleveland to a different city, away from her family, because she was afraid for her life. I remember at about this time, at four years old, I was thinking, *"I need to be responsible, I need to take care"*. My mom told me, *"You have to be a big girl now, you have to grow up and help your mom,"* And I took it very seriously.

We moved to Cincinnati, Ohio and my mom, with three little kids, started her own business. In her mind, she thought—that being a business owner would give her the most flexibility. She thought—if she had her own business, she could be home with us after school. So she got her hair license and started working for one of the most well known stylists in the area. Because of that, she also became pretty well known as well.

Because she wanted to ultimately work from home, she bought a house and opened her home salon. This was the late 70's so she was pretty progressive. A single black woman with three children having the mindset to do this wasn't common. She got her own house because she wanted to be home when her children got home from school. Her home salon became very busy and until she got remarried, that's how it was. I watched her do all of this—and to me, she was a straight-up superhero. In my mind I thought, *"Women are incredible"*. But I also thought that it was hard so I definitely did not want to be a single mother. Please. I didn't want to be a stereotype. I wanted to be educated, get my degree, and marry once to someone for 50 years. I had all these things in my mind and *it* had to be like this.

Anyway, some time later, she got remarried. My stepdad was a good father, a good husband, and a hard-working guy. He came from a rough upbringing, straight up from the streets but was a hard-working guy with a lot of skills in selling. My mom saw that and she talked him into becoming an entrepreneur.

They started their business in the mid-80's. My mom was the one that spearheaded all of *that* and they were very successful in the 80s. They had their own home improvement business and it did well. We moved into a much bigger home. Do you know the theme song from that show, The Jeffersons?, *"Well, We're moving on up?"* That's literally what was going on. They moved into a beautiful home and—I'm watching all this thinking, *"Man, this is how I want it to be. I want to marry once, have a good husband and I want to have my own business with him."* I was also thinking, *"We would do this together and I definitely don't want to be a single mom."* I pushed myself and put myself through college.

Fast forward—After college, I got married the first time and went into corporate america. I pushed myself through college, graduated, started a side business, was making money, and owned investments. Then around 2008, when the economy went down, everything that I had created during that time went down also. I lost everything including my belief. I had seen my mother running for her life with three little kids do some incredible things and that gave me the belief that anything was possible. But as soon as I hit hardship and things did not go my way, I was broken. What had changed? So—one of the reasons I started *Women with Vision* is because I realized it's all *mindset*. In 2008, I lost everything. I lost my business, my job, my husband and my kid could've been taken away from me. It was like—I couldn't even take care of myself anymore. It was amazing how it went from, *"I could do anything, I could literally change the world"* to, *"I can't even wash my face"*. It was like, *"I can't even take care of myself"*.

I found myself sleeping on somebody's couch or sleeping in my car—and it had me wondering, *"How the heck did I get to this place?"* It was crazy how far it went. After doing some personal development work, I finally started to come back around and get my courage, and stamina back. Some people asked how I was able to do all that—I'll talk about that in a minute. After I finally got to, I was starting to realize that it's all *mindset*. All of this can happen if you have your mind right, I thought, *"Well that's what needs to be happening for these women."* We just need to get our mindset right and that's where *Women with Vision* came from.

'Women with Vision' is an underlying thing of, *'come on girl, come on now you can do this'* and *'you can do this girl.'* It's like the thing that I needed when I was going through my roughest time. When I was crying, carrying on, and wondering *why and why me? Why is this not working?* I was paralyzed and I couldn't figure out what to do next—when what I needed was someone to say, *"Come on now girl."* That's where it comes from. It's kind of an *ode* to my mother for *her*—being that woman and having that kind of *mindset*. It's an *ode* to a lot of the women that I met in my life.

It's for all of *us*—to be able to support each other and help one another to get over it. If you go on my Instagram page *'Women with Vision'* and Facebook *'Women with Vision International'*, you'll see a lot of tips about business, personal development, and mindset stuff. Even if you go to my Tam R Luc Instagram page—it's the same thing. You get tips about business but you also have the mindset stuff because—90% is where your mind is. Of course you have done something, it can't just be all into mindset stuff and not do the work. Therefore, continually working on your mindset is how you will be able to create something.

You have to have a vision first and see where you want to go. You can't just be like—*"I wasn't just running around"* just doing any old thing. You have to say, *"Okay, my vision for myself and my life and my family is this—"* For me, my mindset or my vision for my family was—one, I wanted to find a mate who could do this business with me, someone who I love to be a partner with in everything. I wanted to have the vision of being able to empower other women to create the life they wanted to do, and I also envisioned traveling. I didn't want to just work and never get a chance to enjoy my life; part of my enjoyment is traveling and that's part of my business, my life, my lifestyle—and my vision.

When doing a *vision boarding*, come up with what you're going to create in your life. Your vision board could be, *"I want a beautiful house and I want a beautiful car."* Other visions can be, *"I want this certain kind of body. I want to make sure that I go to church weekly, and get involved in giving back to the society."* All those things that are on your vision board are part of your *vision*. Women have to have a *vision*. Then you have to have a way to go forward with that vision. I believe that we all can support each other with our visions while all of us get it.

Supporting each other doesn't mean one of us won't make it. So, supporting each other, collaborating, and connecting is also very important. Then there's this concept of *bossing up*. I spent many years as a side-hustling entrepreneur. In other words, I had my business around my job—I was a side hustler. My very first book that I put out was called *"A Woman's Side Hustle"* and you can get that on Amazon. A *Woman's Side Hustle* came from learning when I was young. My mom taught us how to do what we had to do—to survive. She knew how to do it—she did hair and had these access to all these people.

If someone said, *"I'm going to clean out my cupboards"*, she said, *"My girls can help you"*. If they say, *"I'm looking for somebody to help me clean my house"* her response was, *"My girls can help you"*. *"It's going to be summertime and I'm a teacher, so I need somebody to come and help me straighten out my classroom"*—then again she says, *"My girls can help you"*. My mom was always getting us some kind of side hustle, so we learned how to do it as a young person. All my life I side hustled. Even when I had a job, I was a *side hustler*. That was really just showing you what kind of ideas you can do to side hustle if you need to make that work to survive. That's what side hustling is about.

I spent all those years side hustling when I didn't want to. I wanted to be a full-on boss, have a business where I was making a lot of money like seven figures. I wanted that kind of lifestyle but I couldn't figure out how to do it. Now—my next series is all about *'bossing up'* because finally, I figured out how to do it. It took me some time but I've finally figured out how to *boss up*. Bossing up to me is when you finally jump off that cliff. It is when you finally believe in yourself enough to let go or break away from the umbilical cord.

A lot of side hustling is all about surviving, figuring out what you will and will not do, what you can and cannot do. It's about getting your training, learning how to get clients, how to get a system, and how to be consistent. All that is going on during the side hustle and what happens after that is when you finally boss up, you just break away from that umbilical cord—then you are on your own. You can *boss up* in many ways. Let's say—if you're in a really bad, abusive relationship, you boss up when you finally decide and realize that, *"Look I deserve better than that, I don't want to be in this situation anymore, and I don't deserve to be in the situation,"*—you can boss up.

You can boss up and say, *"You know what, kiss my butt. I'm not staying in this anymore."* You can boss up when you were used to having a certain lifestyle but your husband's lost his job and you have to do something different than you weren't used to doing—that's bossing up and believing in yourself. In that sense, bossing up is believing in yourself and going for what you want. That's the next part after *women who side hustle*, you have to *boss up*.

I'm excited about this new series because I have all these incredible women who have bossed up in so many different ways. That's what they have done in their life and business. Some of them have similar situations and some have different situations. Some have really tragic situations while some have easy. You will find yourself saying, *"If they can do it, I can do it"*. That's the whole point of it. I definitely want you to tune in to this new season. Also in this season, we will have a lot more podcasts coming at you. The goal is to have three per week,

Monday, Wednesday, and Friday. I hope they will not overwhelm you, but there will be a lot of new and amazing women that I want to introduce you to.

I hope that you get so filled up with *possibility*. Right now we're in a very interesting time because there is a pandemic. Some people are feeling like, *"Oh gosh, I was just starting my business, getting clear, ready to go and now—I can't go, I've been stopped, I don't know what to do. I'm thinking I'm going to wait, I'm going to hold off and I'm going to put my head in the sand."* All these things that are going on cause so many emotions, so much fear and you say *"I don't know what's going to happen and how am I going to feed my family?"* There are so many things.

Hopefully this helps you enough to say, *"You know what, if they can do it, I can do it and this is how I can do it."* That's what this is all about, to really empower you to feel you can make this happen for yourself.

Thank you so much for being fans of the Women *with Vision* podcast. I'm so excited that we have kept going. I truly love podcasting. I didn't know I was going to love it so much.

"My strength didn't come from lifting heavy weights, my strength came from lifting myself up every time I was knocked down."

—KARISSA WILLIAMS

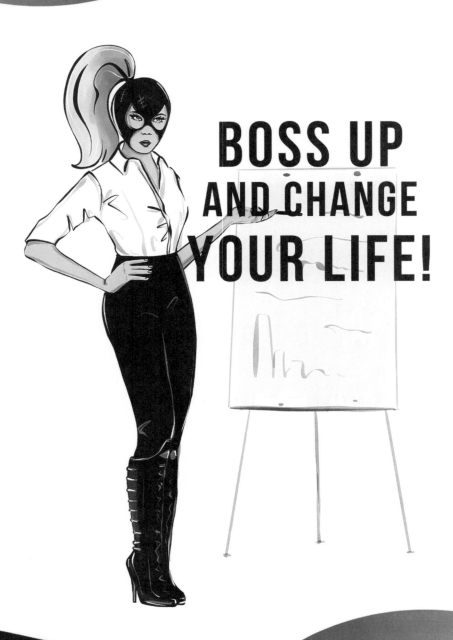

BOSS UP
AND CHANGE
YOUR LIFE!

SECTION 2:
Women Who BossUp in Life

Do you ever think that life should be easier?

Many people are playing too small when it comes to going for what they really want. They're holding back their brilliant ideas and their talents and wasting their time in jobs that just aren't right for them. If you don't listen to your heart, soon enough you will end up burned out, distressed, and disillusioned. You might be in a stable financial situation, but this does not guarantee that you will be satisfied with your life. I want to show you how your life will feel easier and freer when you are working hard at a business you love.

CHAPTER 2:

"Master Your Mind"
with Roma Bajaj Kohli

I AM EXCITED today to introduce my next guest. I met her not that long ago, and she is truly incredible for what she has already created in her life, especially given some of her past experiences. Her name is, Roma Bajaj Kohli.

Q: Roma, what part of the country are you calling from?
New Jersey.

Q: It's difficult right now in New Jersey, right?
Yes, it is.

Q: How is your family doing?
My family's doing great health wise, though they're just about to rip each other apart because we're sitting at home all the time. My husband loves it honestly, but the kids are missing their friends and school.

Q: It's such a new thing, and after so long, you feel like you're bouncing off the walls. Things are so different than what we're used to. I think it's harder for kids.
Yes. Also, outside parks and everything is closed here. Even if they get out, my kids feel like they have nothing to do.

Q: Well, you are a life coach, you're a motivational speaker and you lead a women's empowerment organization in New Jersey. Many people do need to be empowered and they need to be motivated. You didn't start as a coach. So, tell me a little bit about your global traveling adventures.
Right. I'm from India originally and I hadn't previously travelled much by myself or got any opportunity to explore different places because I was born into a very protective family. My parents really wanted to keep me close. I was married at a relatively young age when I was 21 years old. My spouse had a travelling job that allowed us to live in London, Paris, Switzerland, and now the United States. So I was exposed to a lot of different cultures and lifestyles post my marriage.

Q: So, you've been traveling a lot but during that time you were a fashion apparel designer. Did that start in India? Were you in fashion before?

I joined a fashion school when I was in my undergrad right after completing my high school. I knew I was very creative, and I wanted to just explore my imagination and creativity. I worked in India, but it was not until I came to London for the first time, that I realised how diverse, vibrant and exciting this whole industry was. It took me almost forever to get any kind of job in London even though I had earned my diploma in fashion apparel design.

Before I went to London, I was working with a company in India where I was heading the corporate wear brand. When my husband had this opportunity to work in London, I went with him and in the beginning it was so fun until it came time to find something for me to do. It was very hard for me to find any job as most of the places told me that my Indian academic background and fashion apparel designing experience back in India wasn't recognized. They wanted me to either have an MBA or some kind of certification from London itself. To add to our miseries we did not have much clarity at that time about my husband's job duration. So, to commit to a long term course was hard. Though I didn't lose hope and decided to start from scratch and fortunately I landed an internship. It took me about eight to nine months to land a proper job.

But I was only lucky for a very short duration. My work as a Denim wear designer for an export house which created outerwear for high street brands like Topshop, River Island, and Zara was exciting as well as fulfilling and the company's culture was great, but I was in that job for about 6 months. Due to the 2008 recession, my husband's job duration was cut short and his assignment in London came to an abrupt end! The economy had hit an all time low..It was almost like overnight we had to pack our entire lives there and travel back to India. When we returned to India, I wanted to have my own identity and independence. Yet I didn't want to go back to my previous job, as my perspective had changed and I wanted to contribute in a much more meaningful way to the fashion world. I was intrigued by the exposure of the global fashion world that I got in London. So every time we moved from a location, I got an opportunity to re-evaluate who I wanted to be then. Which used to seem like a curse back then was actually my biggest blessing! My views and perspective of life kept on growing and I kept on consistently evolving. Both as an individual and on a professional and spiritual level.

Q: This is so good because not everyone is so self-aware. When you went back to India, what did you decide?

Luckily we went back to my home city of Pune. We had our parents, and our home there. But, there weren't as many fashion and design houses there at that time. And as I said before I was longing this time for something more. Then I was a bit overwhelmed with confusion. I am a typical type A personality. Out of nowhere one day I got a text from one of my old professors. He was teaching at a well renowned design institute and I was talking to him about how I wanted to do something more. He told me that there is an opportunity for teaching global fashion communication and history of fashion in the design school where he was and asked me to meet with the Head of the department (HOD) there. He said, "Why don't you just apply to see if you can get a teaching job there." And I'm like, "No, I haven't ever taught before." I'm way too young" or just two or three years older than my students at that time so how can I teach them?

Nevertheless with all my inhibitions, fears and skepticism I went ahead for an interview. The HOD was a very nice person. Apart from the fact that I got the job I became a teacher at 23 years old. And just doing that work lifted my spirits up to a whole new dimension. I loved every bit of my life then. The global experience of starting from scratch and going through the internship phase all over again and working in London, gave me the confidence to deconstruct and reconstruct. I wasn't attached to any ego of who I was and what I did. My students loved me just as much I loved them. I started mentoring and coaching degree project students for final year submissions. I hadn't even realised how passionate I was for teaching and guiding my students. Then my husband got a great opportunity to work in Zurich, Switzerland and we decided to leave given his future prospects.

Q: That is incredible. You're now teaching at a university. When you get to Switzerland, what happens?
I mean, as much as I was enjoying my life as a professor the hunger to travel and see the world was way more exciting for me. So even though learning the local

language "german" was a challenge in itself and all that settling in was definitely challenging and would make me question our desires to keep relocating and travelling. But I think I was young and I want you to see the world because I had never really gotten a chance earlier to explore different places. It felt like we were on our extended honeymoon and we're enjoying our adventures! As usual it took me about six months to find something to do worthwhile there. A friend of mine who had his own private label that time, has reached out to me as he found me on social media and figured that I was in Europe. He has a brand called GOPE in West Bengal, India. He would digitally design the Batik prints and the artisans would produce the same design by hand dyeing and hand weaving the fabrics.

His work was very intriguing to me. He told me he was coming to Paris, to exhibit his collection at PRET-A-PORTER Paris and if I'd want to come and help him there, and I was like, "of course!" it's a dream come true for every fashion designer to be in the PRET-A-PORTER exhibition. I was going no matter what. So he shipped his entire collection of clothes and accessories to me.

Q: Gorgeous.

So, I headed to Paris with his stuff 2 days before the show. I got to travel and see Paris as a tourist. One night before the show was about to start, he told me he couldn't make it because the Indian embassy did not approve his Schengen visa. And that was it! I was so freaked out with fear and anxiety. I mean, was I supposed to sell his collection. I felt like I didn't know much about it. I don't even know his business that well. I thought I was just going to help him out in the set-up etc. He tried to cancel the show but as he had paid everything upfront one day before, there was no way to get a cancellation. So after all the panic was over I surrendered and took some basic training from him about his collection and went on my own to set-up the show and I surprised myself yet again.

It was very interesting, the people I met, and the subsequent business I secured for his brand. I didn't even know that I was so good at building relationships with people and making sales. I never experienced that before and this was my first exposure to living the life of an *Entrepreneur*.

Looking back I feel fortunate enough that all these events and so called challenges in my life have become one of the most awesome teaching and evolving mile-stones. Those situations have made me realise my true self and tapped into my resilient nature. It revealed my true identity to me and brought forward my many superpowers. Isn't it true that adversity is the greatest teacher of all times!

Q: You are a "yes". That has given you all these experiences that many people do not have because they are not in that "Yes" space. You could have been like, no, I can't do that. I'm not good enough. You could have easily said no when you were invited to interview for that job to be a faculty member. It tells a lot about you. That's amazing.
It was very shocking for me as well. I mean all those giant leaps were so scary at that time, yet looking back

and connecting those dots I can totally see how it has shaped me and my life and the work I do today!

Q: How long were you partners with this guy?
I worked with him for about two years and I had also given birth to my first child during this time and the hours were getting a bit taxing and eventually I gave up the partnership.

Q: Did you become a coach at that point? Did you decide that you wanted to do a switch or were you still in the fashion industry?
When I was in Switzerland, I was still looking for full time jobs in the fashion industry, but with my child at home, I was finding it hard to take that much time off in case I landed up a job. I wanted something I could work part-time from home or full time from home. It took me about a year. to find something. Though I did study German for two levels there, even then, I was still managing only basic level German. Which i knew wasn't really taking me too far. As I was adjusting to become a new mom, I landed a job with Esprit. I was their catalog designer. I would just take pictures of their garments on mannequin and then do the flat layouts for their monthly catalogues. Again, that worked for six months and that was it. It was time for us to come back to India. Our work permit to be in that country has expired. So, it was challenging.

I won't paint the picture, saying I traveled almost half of the world and it was easy for me to just figure everything out. It wasn't, I've had my share of and just feeling like *why has life been so unkind?* When I connected the dots back, I realized that all those adventures, and challenges made me the guide and coach I'm today!

Q: You created a method which I find very interesting. You're the founder of The Awakened Mind Method, which is an eight-week transformation program for soul-centered women leaders to master their mind by owning their true power and awakening their innate intelligence through play. How did you come up with that?

When I came back to India luckily, I got my job back as the Assistant Professor in the same design school in Pune. Within a couple of months of being in India, my husband got another opportunity to be in New York! This was a bit early for me as I was settling in with my design school again and just being back from Switzerland, I told my husband I think you should just go alone to New York for some time and *(maybe)* I will join later. I just wanted to give myself a little bit of time and honor the commitment I gave to my college when I got the job back again. He was fine with it as I was in Pune and said, *okay, fine.* I was enjoying my teaching job back at the university and they wanted me to become a permanent faculty. I was considering that and I wanted to stick with my career now. I wanted more consistency and stability in my career. Though just about six months after he left, I was like, *I can't do this.* My child was missing his bonding of being with his dad and it was hard on my husband too. So *(once again)* I left my full time job back in India and came to the US knowing that I was putting my teaching career at stake for the family.

Then we lived happily ever after! Nah. I was joking. Just a few months after being in the states, that passion of doing something on my own again crept up.

I was like a serial entrepreneur. I would sleep with business ideas in my head. I would wake up with them and then I would cry and just throw them in the trash by myself. I didn't know what to do. When I say I help women tap into their innate intelligence, through play, what I mean is that doing what I love was my playtime. I was so sick and tired of taking all the emotional, mental, and physical pressure that everytime I would see my kids play so freely at the park, I was able to see how happy, joyful and present they were. It was in some of those moments that I decided that those are the feelings I wanted to create for myself! I knew that I wanted to be my own boss. But I I didn't know what and how. So, after a lot of soul searching and putting together all my life experiences, yoga certifications, lifestyle coaching degrees and so on. I developed The Awakened Mind framework.

We need to make sure we are working on all aspects of our being. Starting with Mindset Revival to the physical aspect of Mindful Movement, learning to manage and master our emotions through Breakthrough Breathwork, while taking care of our food and bringing harmony and balance in our lives through Visualisation Meditation. I help my clients bring all aspects of their personal and professional lives in balance through play.

Q: It's true. I was watching this program the other day about getting things done and being more productive and they say that to be more productive, it should be like playing.

Yes.

Q: You are more creative at play. People are not even as motivated by money when it comes to creativity.

Yes. 100 percent.

Q: It's all about having fun and you come up with better ideas. What do you think is your biggest hurdle that you've had to overcome?

The biggest hurdle has been the four years of being a stay at home mom and being in the state of a 'Confusedpreneur'. I was known as the 'Confusedpreneur' in my networking group of women, the one that I'm leading now because I used to hate to say that I'm a stay-at-home mom so I coined that term up for me. I think that's the hardest thing to do right now.

My biggest hurdle was those four years of figuring out what I love to do. As a mom, I knew the value of time and energy. I was spending time with my kids. I had to do something as substantial and impactful, that would not make me feel guilty for taking the time away from my kids. I think that was my hardest and biggest hurdle.

And COVID has bought those fears back because the first week my kids were back from school and I just felt like, *Oh, my God, am I getting sucked into the same spiral?* And the fear of being that stay at home mom again was totally showing up in my business. I felt like

I had just learned to walk the fine line of balancing and I was just mastering the art of being aware and conscious of my time and managing my days optimally and that was when COVID happened. And then I'm like, everyone's home, everyone's constantly hungry. Kids constantly need me for their remote learning. And I was like just tearing my head apart.

As a mom of 2 young kids I think, your audience would love to hear this, the third day into the COVID, I cried and I just gave up and I told my husband, I want you to have an adult conversation. So, I said to the kids, *can you please excuse us?* And I cried my heart out to my husband and said, to him `*Do you think this awakened mind method, the online program that I'm about to launch, should push it back for a few months*`?

After much thinking and contemplation my husband and I agreed, and he said, yeah, looks like this is a very stressful time for everyone because obviously, the fear was getting onto him as well. And so, he was like, yeah, I think I agree you should push it back. I almost made peace with the fact that instead of launching in May, I will launch it in a few more months and that would give me a breather to adjust with the kids and stuff.

I came out of my discussion with my husband and my daughter who is a very curious child (she's seven!) asked me, "Mommy what were you and Daddy talking about?" And I have been very open and honest with my kids. I told them that mom has pushed her programme's launch date back. My son who is 9 was listening to some audio books and I cannot forget his expression. He was sitting on the kitchen island

and when I said to my daughter that Papa and I have decided that I will push back my work, because it's just too much to manage with all of you at home. My son just closes his laptop with his eyes wide open and he says, *"No, no, no, no, no, no. That is not happening."*

Q: That is hilarious.
He said to me, *"Are you pushing your work back for us? If that's something we need to figure out that's between Aarna and me, we'll figure it out.* Just like Daddy gets eight hours of work, you will be given three to four hours in the daytime from us. Free to do whatever you need to do. You can isolate yourself. You can sit in the room wherever you want, but that's not happening. You are not pushing your work behind. One more time."

Q: I love this kid.
I just froze. My body was like, yes, these are the humans I produced in this world.

Q: These are the humans that you created. I cannot get enough of that. I wish that were on video. I would play that every single day. That is the best thing ever.
As a mom or as an individual we all are looking for that one push, that one permission, that unwavering faith and belief in ourselves and imagine how elevating and uplifting this whole experience can be if your little kids become that for you!

I mean I knew that this is it. What I'm so proud of is that I'm leaving a legacy of kindness and empathy behind. We were celebrating in the kitchen, and my husband comes up, and he's like, *"What's this commotion?*

Your mother was crying 10 minutes ago and now you guys are like, music is on everyone's dancing. What just happened?" And my son said, *"We gave Mamma the time and space to keep doing her business. 'WOW!' my husband said. 'So, my son says 'you see papa you and Mumma didn't make a very smart decision'.* And my husband was like, "That's all. That's it. If you guys can support us, there's so much we can do, be and achieve as a family."

Q: This is everything. This is my philosophy. Women are like spaghetti. Everything touches. We don't compartmentalize things as well because everything touches. So for it to work you have to include your family into the process. So they understand what's happening, then they're rooting for you. It was so smart of you to include them because he gave you the best advice ever.
Right.

Q: I think everyone should look at it like that and not use their kids as an excuse.
For me, my business only started because of my kids. I just want to leave a legacy behind they would be proud of.

Q: You talked about the Awakened Mind and you might have it in your programme, but what do you use to be motivated and stay in the game?
I must tell you that coaching wasn't always a part of my life. But ever since I think I was five or six, I always said that when I grow up, I want to be Mother Teresa. Then I got introduced to Oprah Winfrey. I mean, we all want to be her. I said I wanted to be her. I wanted to

do what she does. I realized that they were all teachers, guides and inspirations. I always wanted to do that.

For me, my motivation comes from the fact that now I have taken a hundred percent responsibility for who I am and who I want to become. Just simply being in alignment and integrity and congruence with myself is what motivates me. I don't just do this for me or money. I do it because I have these little human's watching me everyday and every night.

Every morning when we wake up, my daughter, she looks up to me as the woman of the house and she looks at me whether I'm happy and when I'm not. You know how kids are, they usually pick up the mother's energy. Even now, my kids are nine and seven. They still pick up my energy. If I'm having a fabulous, mentally, happy day, they are happy. If not, they get cranky along with me. For me, doing something, even two hours, three hours of daily work, I put in myself and my business gives me so much happiness and contentment. They see that in me. My lightness, the energy in me, that lights up their eyes.

Q: What advice would you give to anyone going through something, or they're where they're feeling stuck? They are in COVID 19 and they're feeling down about the situation. Is there any advice you would give to an entrepreneur?

Yeah, I mean, I would just tell them that COVID 19 cannot bring up any unknown fears. It will only bubble on the surface what is already existing within you. If your fears are larger than they were ever before it's totally understandable. Yet you choose in this moment who gets to be in the driver's seat - Your intelligence or Your fear? I mean only you can hold your hand and walk through the other side of the bridge. As much as I want to say that my kids helped me make that decision, the real reason I shared it with my kids was deep down inside me. I kind of knew that the decision which my husband and I made didn't feel right. Because I was like, push it back until when? None of us know when COVID was ending. You don't have an end date, there is so much unknown in the future. So what I have is the NOW.

I lead a women's empowerment organization, I hear the woman saying all the time, *Oh no, no. This is not a time to sell.* This is just a time to give freebies and I'm like, *do you know why you sell?* If you sell to serve for the highest purpose, and good you don't even need to worry about what is the right time . Every moment is right.

Q: Every moment is right. Because we are servants of the lord.
Yes.

Q: We have a service. No matter what, we are here to help. What we have created, what we have overcome, what we have with the transformation that we've gotten, we are here and that transforms other people. So, we are servants. If you are always in that mindset, there is never a wrong time to give that and you should be compensated for that.
Thank you.

Q: So if you want to learn more about Roma, go to her website www.wellnessbyroma.com or on instagram @wellnessbyroma, stay connected with her. Thank you so much, Roma.

Thank you, Tam truly. It is a pleasure to know you and be part of this amazing tribe!

"Uncovering your authenticity is a way to re-claim your essence, your power, your value, your worth—and from that place, you can create the life you have always wanted."

—JENNIFER BLAIR

CHAPTER 3:

"Balance, purpose, and passion"
with Jennifer Blair

HEY THERE, SUPERWOMEN. I am really excited to have my next guest today hailing from Louisville, Kentucky to share her story.

> **Q: Jennifer Blair, welcome.**
> Thank you so much. I'm thrilled to be here. Thanks for having me.

Q: You are a leading life coach, inspirational speaker, and author from Louisville, Kentucky. You received your training from the Coactive Training Institute, and you then went on to create your company. Can you tell me a little about that, what led you to start your coaching business, and what you do now?

Okay. Well, I can't believe I'm in my 17th year—wow—and still going strong, still loving it. I'll go further than that to give you some background. I moved here from Dallas, Texas in 1990 to get married, expecting to be a wife, a mother, create a family, that sort of thing. I had been working in corporate America. I was doing big communication projects for a company in Dallas called EDS, and moving to Louisville, I found the companies here just don't work that way.

So, when I had my first child, my husband and I decided that I would become a stay-at-home mom. That was awesome at the beginning, and I was so grateful for the opportunity, but I also quickly realized how difficult it is to be at home by yourself with a baby or toddler. So, I got myself extremely involved with volunteer work, had another child, and did that for ten years. However, around year nine, my marriage started to fall apart, and it finally blew up. We got into marriage counseling, and I read all types of books, got into individual therapy, trying to figure out what was going on, and what was happening to my life. After two years, I decided to leave the marriage.

What I haven't mentioned is that I had a very big community role at the time. I was the president of the Junior League of Louisville in our 80th anniversary year. When I made the decision to divorce, it was quite shocking to people because no one knew that I had these issues going on at home. I was one of these people that kept it to myself and didn't ask for help. I can vividly remember standing at the podium at a Junior League meeting somewhere in the spring of that year, looking out at a hundred or so women, and thinking, "How many other women sit in silence and suffer and never speak up about what's going on with their lives. They don't reach out for support or help. I couldn't be the only one, could I?"

So, I decided to get a divorce, and I spent a couple of years healing— I didn't want to be one of these bitter, wounded, and angry women. I kept thinking I would write a book on divorce and while I was in a bookstore looking for books on this topic, and one day I ran across a book called Live Your Best Life by Laura Berman Fortgang, and in it she said, "Therapy heals the past, coaching moves you forward." I thought, "That's it! I don't know what coaching is, but I am doing that— something to move myself and others forward in life." So, I bought the book, came home and within three weeks, I found the Coaches Training Institute, which is now the Co-Active Training Institute, and I signed up for my first training. I was in the summer of 2003, and I did a fast track of coaches training. My thinking was that I don't want to just write a book only about my divorce experience. So, I might as well interview other women, and if I'm doing that, I might as well help heal them and work with them.

This is how I came to create my business. I did my coaching training and a few other training around intuition, transformation, and some spiritual training as well. I came up with the name Excavive, which means to excavate your life. So, I created my brand and hung up the sign that said, "I'm in business."

Q: There are so many things I'm pulling from this. Most coaches, life coaches, or any kind of coach probably started from something blowing up.
Yes, absolutely.

Q: Something had to blow up, something had to not be working right. And when you hit the fork in the road where you're saying this is not working, and then you make the change.
Absolutely, and I think the biggest thing I realized out of that, which I really want others to hear and maybe understand, is that it wasn't just that my life blew up and things weren't going to be the same. The biggest motivation for me getting out of that marriage was the realization that I had lost sight of who I was. I had to get back to who I am, and, like a phoenix rising from the ashes, be bolder, stronger, and fiercer, to go do what I need to do in the world, whatever that may be. I realized that every painful thing in life I go through is meant to be healed, to transform me into something great.

Q: I love this because your life looked a certain way to everyone else who was watching. But underneath, it's all different. Sometimes people don't want to get past it and do the work. They'll just say I don't want anyone else to know, and then they suffer in silence.
This is absolutely the case. You know, I wasn't only the Junior League president— I had been the chair of 'The

Race for the Cure,' I was on the board of the Science Center, I co-chaired things at my children's school, and I co-chaired the largest, most prestigious fundraiser, The Speed Art Museum Ball. I had this very public persona, and I looked the part. I used to say I should win an Academy Award for the role I was playing. And you know, I had my house, my two little children, my attorney husband, and I would get dressed up in my beautiful clothes, jewelry, and makeup, then walk out into the world and look like life couldn't be better, right? But inside I was dying, and I was suffering in silence. Not only that, but the only people that I could talk to about this situation were back in Texas because I wanted to make sure that it didn't get back across the border into Kentucky. For a long time, these were the only people who knew anything about what was going on with me. Until it reached a breaking point when I needed to do something.

Q: Yes, how many other women are like that? You were standing there thinking I'm probably not the only one.

Well yes, I was sure there had to be others like me—there had to be! So, I went through a fairly public divorce, and it was amazing to me how many people who knew us were saying, "I had no idea." And how other women started to reach out to me. That was one way I knew I was right to start this business because people would say, "I'm having some trouble too, would you? I need someone to talk to." I think that is one of the reasons I've been in business for 17 years, that I have a personality, a kind of warmth that people trust. Maybe it's that southern Texas part of me, which allows people to connect with me and the other way around.

Q: Fantastic. So, you've been in business for 17 years now. You've seen plenty. What do you think are the biggest hurdles that you've had to overcome?

Great question. People often assume it must be tough listening to people's problems all day long, hearing about the suffering, but to be honest, that's not the hard part for me. I have some phenomenal tools I use to take care of myself. I think what was difficult to overcome was learning about the ebb and flow of business. The highs of abundance, which could be amazing, and the lows, when money's not flowing, which could be really tough. It took me years to build that inner resilience and strength and to truly understand that I was going to be all right no matter what.

I always said I had faith, but to really believe that, I had to put a lot of tools in place for myself, like journaling and meditation as well as being fierce to do the work and to look after yourself. Self-care has to be part of the business plan. You have to get into the space of believing and taking action because coaching is the easy part. I have this term, "sustained believability," which is my ability to keep going. It's faith and inspired action combined, deep, deep, faith in myself and in God to keep showing up every day. My job is to stay grounded and positive and to live what I teach others. To do this can get scary, but you just tell someone this and get up and do it anyway, again and again.

Q: I think this is the best way to live. It's the mindset of a boss, you know? Bossing up. It's being scared and doing it anyway.

Absolutely, and the reason I call it sustained is because it doesn't mean I don't get those moments of fear; it's that I keep going anyway. Right now, this time of COVID-19 is a great example. We are just being hit on the head with fear, and I keep coming back to my tools, my faith, my meditation, and I sit down and do the work. I follow up with clients, I ask for the money, I keep doing it, and I show up every day.

Q: That's right. Can you give me another obstacle or challenge that came up for you? Other than right now with COVID-19.

Well, I'll go all the way back to my childhood. My parents divorced when I was 13 years old, and my dad was an alcoholic. I grew up with that; certainly, my mother and grandmother were very supportive, but it was a very difficult time. I took on the traits of the child of an alcoholic; co-dependency was something I really had to work very hard on. You don't feel very deserving, that you are not or haven't done enough. Taking that into adulthood and then having a marriage fall apart, which only reinforced it, was one of the biggest things I've had to overcome. I'm 57 now.

Q: You look beautiful, by the way. When you told me that last time, I thought you're crazy, you are not 57.

You're so sweet. The only reason I mention it is because it took me until I was in my early 50s, even though I was a coach and I had this business, to overcome this obstacle of feeling like I deserved this— that I was enough, and I could make a living coaching people and also deserved to receive abundance. I think it goes back to growing up in an alcoholic home with divorced parents. My parents divorced, mom did not even have a college education, so she went back to school, got her interior design degree, and started her own business, even with two small children. She just did it, and I saw that. That was a great example, so I thought maybe I can do it too.

Q: Right. I think that is common to a lot of people. I had to deal with a little of that. I think that's kind of part of being human; am I enough? It usually comes up early in life, from our parents or some kind of situation, where it's kind of drilled in early.
Absolutely.

Q: And you've become self-aware enough to turn it around.
Absolutely. I really believe that these experiences, I now call them "transformational opportunities" have grown me and given me an enormous opportunity to truly transform, to change myself for the better—be it divorce, or a child of divorce, or many other challenges, I can name many, many others. So, every experience I have, I can turn around and use with my clients and with the people who read my books. I feel that they're not my experiences to hold onto any longer, that I have to put them back out there for others so they can learn as well.

Q: Yeah. You've mentioned different things you do to stay focused and your tools, but you like to do fun stuff as well. Can you tell me about that?

Well, having arrived where I have given myself permission to have this amazing life, over the last 17 years, I've really embraced the things that make me happy and gotten back into things I'm passionate about or feel deeply connected to. I try to live a balanced life, to take care of myself with things like Pilates, walking, massages, journaling, and meditating— I love my downtime. But I also really engage in things I love, like travel, art, and beauty. I love them; they're huge motivators for me. I take lots of classes in flower arranging, and I do that a lot. I'm dating a man who said he'll always supply me with flowers. I think he got my heart when he said that, and every week or so, he brings me fresh flowers, which I then get to arrange. I love to cook, salsa dance, and I write for my business. For inspiration, I read lots. I'm in a book club where we read just fiction, which is a nice break from self-help books. I also believe in cultural outings, so I'm very involved in the Speed Art Museum and am on the Board of Governors. I joined their Contemporary Collector's Group, so I get to go on trips to amazing places like Mexico City last year and Cleveland and Los Angeles the year before.

I love nature and getting out in nature. It keeps me motivated and grounded, to observe what's happening in the world. Because we're all stuck at home now, I like to stay in touch with people, not by email or texting, but by calling and actually speaking with them. I do that every day— go for a walk, connect with others and take the time to just feel everything. I allow the emotions to come, even the fears, so I can let them dissipate, and they don't have a hold on me. I acknowledge them, but I don't hold on to them. So, I stay motivated in lots of ways, but the main one is my clients. They have entrusted me with their journeys, and they motivate me each and every day, and I have such gratitude for that and to see them transform.

Q: I love that. What would you say to entrepreneurs from your 17 years' experience? What advice can you give them?

It's interesting you asked me this question because I do some inspirational speaking, and I've seen my topics change over the years, but I've recently been tapped to talk about "Stepping Up Your Success." I've been thinking about what it takes to be successful over and over and over again, and I've come up with my five keys to it. Number one is you've got to "love what you do;" you've got to really love it. You have to be emotionally determined to do it. Number two is "cultivated clarity." I think you've got to really cultivate and be very clear with yourself what success looks like for you. Why are you doing it, who are you best serving? It's got to be reciprocal in that you get as much out of it as you put in. Number three is "confident believability." You have to really believe that you can do it when you pick your path. I've seen so many clients come to me and they want to change their lives, careers whatever, and they gradually fade. You have to dig deep down and connect to that believability. Number four is "empowered action." You've got to match desire and believability with action. I tell people to pick three things a day to do, five days a week—that's 60 actions a month. If you're doing that, you have to make progress. Number five is "sustained self-care and support." Give yourself permission to be replenished and re-fueled. That's my five, but I think it's believability (in themselves or their dreams) that people sometimes lack the most.

Q: They do. I see a lot of that, too. And you have a new book. Can you tell me a little about that?
In 2011, I published a book called The True You that was a compilation of columns I'd written for a local magazine called Underwired. At the time, it was a marketing tool to sell at the back of the room when I was giving talks, and it did well. It sold lots and led to great things. Last summer, my publishing company approached me to do another edition, so I decided to take that, and I'm calling the new book The True You Reimagined: Discover Your Authentic Self. I took the best of what was there and reworked it, added a new section that is career related. I'm creating this book that is all about what it takes to uncover your authenticity and reclaim who you are. It has lots and lots of tools and coaching questions in it and is divided into six sections and will be out at the beginning of June. In fact, I'm sending it to the publishers, hopefully by this Friday, and I'm super excited about it. I'm also working on The True You Workbook: Tools to Reimagine Your Life, which will go with it. Over my 17 years, I've created about 45 coaching exercises, and they're going in the workbook to use alongside the book or separately. The format of the book, The True You Reimagined, is I give the reader a coaching perspective and a helpful list

because sometimes people don't like to read. They prefer a quick list of topics or bullet points. And every chapter has a couple of coaching questions at the end— I think it's important to invite the reader to become involved in what I'm talking about. I don't just want to talk to some-body. So, the intention is to really bring you the reader into it and help you be your best, the best version of who you are, and what you're up to in the world.

Q: Well, I love it, I love everything that you're doing. How can we stay connected to you? Give us your website.

My website is www.excavive.com, and if you go and sign up for my email list, I have a free e-book called Be Who You Are: Six Steps to Excavate Yourself. You can sign up right on the homepage, and you'll get a copy of the e-book immediately.

Q: I love it. Jennifer, you are a joy. I'm so glad that we met, and we are going to be doing lots of collabora-tions in the future. Thank you so much, and it's been amazing having you on.

Thank you so much. This has been a thrill to meet you and be on your show. I look forward to what we're going to be up to together in the next few months.

"Spend time adding to your cup and give time for yourself."

—TAM LUC

CHAPTER 4:

"Look Up, Reach Out and Step Forward"
with Life Coach Kimberley Loska

KIMBERLEY LOSKA HAS been motivating audiences as a coach, training leaders, doing workshops, and hosting retreats for the last 20 years. She helps people find purpose in the pain and I'm so excited to hear all about her story.

Q: How did you start off coaching?
I think some of us, when we finally find our lane, it's

coming to the place of realization. I've been doing this since I was a little girl, when you really get down to it. This is my heartbeat. This is what gets the juices flowing for me. Honestly, it's to bring people to a place where they can recognize the boss within them. It's always been there but sometimes we go through a few rodeos before we can recognize it.

Q: What are some of those circumstances that came up early in life?
Early in life, my parents divorced. I was from a Mayberry kind of town, typical of California. Divorce wasn't something that was really done, and it was my first taste of reality. Trauma is going to come to all of us to some degree, but what do we do with it? What do we lean on when that impact happens in our life? Later we moved from Crescent City, California, to Summerland near Santa Barbara. My life took a total turn because everything was new. It's not about who is around us, but what is within us that makes the difference. That is how we can ride out that storm.

This is such a good question because my first lesson came from my father who never told me he loved me till I was 16. He was very conservative. So, I bumped around with the Daddy-doesn't-love-me syndrome. I bumped around in high school. Picture this. They called me Olive Oil because I was so skinny, no hips, no booty, nothing. I was a tomboy and felt I had a lot to prove. During that time in high school, I went through a lot. I messed around with drugs, alcohol, and boys. I got pregnant and had an abortion. I was a hot mess.

But there was always that quiet voice in my heart.

There was always that light calling me home. Just a knowing deep within saying: *What are you doing? This isn't who you really are.* But because there was such a lack of mentorship in my life, I guess I had to bump around a bit.

Q: Do you think you experienced some of those things because you are meant to lead others?
Yes. Fast forwarding, I've always been that leader. There are a lot of people who get pretty enamored with themselves, but I like to say that I was always very well grounded in the sense that I knew what I was and wasn't. When I was 20 years old, I met a guy I thought was all of that and a bag of chips. He was like a knight in shining armor. So charming that he swept me off my feet. It took years for me to learn that he was a complete narcissist.

I was a perfect magnet for a narcissist at the time, and we stayed married for 28 years and had three kids. At 20, I was an instant mom. He came with a child from another marriage and I had my first child five years later. He had an amazing mind, a genius IQ, and he became a very successful attorney. I, in-turn, focused my energy on the many women who came into my life.

Because I didn't have a mentor to train me in the basics in life, I became that for other women. I knew I was a strong person, but at the time I wasn't able to embrace everything God had for me. So, I had a huge passion to be that for someone else.

This is why I am called to help women. Women are like a chain-link fence. Each link may look like nothing, but together it's a force to be reckoned with. I started seeing myself as this person, pouring myself into the lives of these other women so they could believe that.

Q: When you were married, did you see problems throughout your marriage or did you not realize it until much later?

Yes. I saw it right away. About three years into our marriage, he was just so jealous and controlling. Much later I realized he had traits of a narcissist and also had borderline personality disorder. This ultimately is like a black hole. You can try to feed it but you can never feed it enough. As I continued in the marriage, I found my voice getting quieter and my bulb was getting more and more dim. It's almost like he was taking my energy to catapult himself forward. I saw a lot of problems, but I came from a divorced family. My mom was married three times, my dad was married three times, my stepdad was married three times, and my stepmom was married three times. So I guess the third time's the charm. I stayed because I thought, *I'm going to be the one that breaks that pattern. I'm going to stick by my man. I'm going to persevere in this marriage.* Even though I became more and more unhappy.

Q: I can relate. How do you feel you lost your voice?

After, the first 10 years of marriage, he confessed to me that he was addicted to pornography. So, once again, I didn't think I was worth anything. This little girl let her voice get smaller and smaller, getting lost in another person's identity. And now I have to compare myself to a woman in porn? It was absolutely awful. It ripped me to the core. Those old voices of not being good enough kept coming at every turn.

So fast forward from there. He says he got help for his addiction then he goes into ministry. We were both leading bible studies in our home and got deeply involved. I was ministering to women who had felt the effects of pornography in their marriage, and he was helping the men. There was a lot of victory there. It was awesome…for a minute.

Then he says he's feeling called to minister to people further. Long story short, he decides to become a pastor of a pretty well-known nondenominational church. We started a church in our barn that really evolved. We started with six people one weekend, and it became a movement.

We led it together for 10 years. We had very famous pastors in our house on a regular basis and a talk on a radio show that was heard far and wide. I really thought, *God is turning this man around.* I saw this new awakening in him.

It was at the end of the 10-year mark that those old compulsions he had fought for so many years took him over. The last eight years of our marriage, he never touched me physically. Once again, we were in another tough rodeo.

He stepped down from the ministry and, six months later, finally confessed he was having an affair with multiple women. Just like that, the bottom dropped out again. I felt like I had lost everything.

He got into alcohol heavily along with cocaine. He was really a mess. For years, we tried to be the billboard couple. We tried counseling. But it did come to the point where I recognized one night that we were done. He left town, and I was left holding the bag—very common for us women. I had to face the community we raised our family in, where he was a very successful attorney and ran a church.

One day at about three o'clock in the morning, I smelled a fragrance in my room and it woke me up. I heard this voice in my heart: *"I'm with you and I'm for you."* I woke up my daughter. *"Did you hear that?"* She said no.

Two more times it came, and by the third time I knew right away. I knew that was the voice of my Lord. When you're suffering, 20 years is a long time. You're like, *Do you not see what's going on?* Tears were streaming down my face. I just said out loud, "I vote for me." And I was done. It was through that process, honestly, that I recognized I had lost myself. I lost my voice and my identity. That is my heart's cry. For other women, I want them to know I've gone through the fire. Sometimes we need somebody to be our voice until we find it again.

Through this process, I learned that what you are going through right now is all relative. Your perception is your reality. But just because it's your perception, that doesn't make it true. My perception was that I'd lost everything. But it was his downward spiral I was feeling for myself until I decided, *No, no, no. This experience is what's going to bring me back to who I really am.*

Pain is a constant, but we have to recognize the purpose in it. What is the purpose in my pain? This is not the end of the story. For me, it was the beginning of doing what I was always meant to do. What I was always supposed to be. So, my purpose now and since I was a little girl, is to lift other women to reach higher ground. And if my pain, my story, and the things I went through preserve a piece of your chain-link fence, then that's what I'm all about. I found that I had to look at that which was higher, because I couldn't figure this out. The second step was to reach out.

Q: I know through your story that things have been up and down. But now, how do you stay motivated?

Well, I will tie the end of the story in with how I stay motivated. John and I divorced. Three years later, he got so lost in his life and lifestyle, he went crazy. He had a mental disorder. He was going to get fired from his job, and he called me the night before and said, "Hey, I've got to talk to you. I'm going to get fired and it's going to impact the kids and you, but I want you to know I love you and I always have." And I said, "Okay, John." Then I said, "You're going to be fine. Everything's going to be fine." But the next day, he went to work with a gun, and he shot and killed his senior partner. He critically injured his other partner, then turned the gun on himself and committed suicide.

So, how does one stay motivated? And the other question is, what does one do when the bottom drops out? I cannot look at John. I cannot look at another person. I cannot look at the circumstances. I cannot look at the house, the car I drive. How do I stay motivated? It's knowing who I am. It's knowing my true identity. I talk a lot about that in my conferences about the identity crisis. Because if we don't know who we are in Christ, we don't know our value. We don't know our worth. If we know our worth, then we don't know our purpose. I have found my purpose. What motivates me is what I see in the faces of other women when they finally hit through that tape. When they bust through with their chest, they persevere. They keep pressing, even when it's hard. Because I'm a life coach, I get to see these breakthroughs every day. It's my purpose. You've got to keep finding, keep digging. You've got to keep availing yourself to transformation because none of us have arrived. If somebody in your life tells you they've arrived, run like your hair's on fire because none of us have arrived and we're constantly being transformed. So, when I see a breakthrough in the life of another woman, that's what spurs me on to do good work. I can shine a light in her life and put a mirror to her face and say, "This is who you are, baby girl. This is who you were always meant to be. It's got that light bulb and it's a little clouded. It doesn't have to stay that way."

Q: Now, let me just be clear. Somebody may be out there in a really bad situation just trying to figure out how to get to the next step. Hopefully, they're inspired by your story. There is always a transformation on the other side of a story, if you choose to have a transformation. So, as a life coach, what do you hope to do?
I did this for a long, long time and was never paid a dime. Money's attached to coaching, for sure. But I've got rent to pay. I've got food I have to buy. And the thing is, I show up with excellence with every single one of my clients because they deserve it. So, we have to look

under the hood and find out. If everything gets blown up, there're pieces everywhere. What do you do? Put it all back together again and it becomes more beautiful.

Japan has a beautiful culture. They never waste anything. When there's a broken bowl, what the artists will do is take this bowl and glue it back together again. Then they layer it with precious gold over the top for all the world to see. The broken pieces bring out even more beauty.

In my book that I'm finishing up, I write about the art of breaking. There is something to it because God redeems brokenness. He loves it. I love this illustration because we want to hide what we think is not perfect and good. We want it to be repaired so that nobody knows it was broken.

The transformation needs to be something we're not embarrassed by. It needs to be something that projects us to the next level. I'm not going to be ashamed of the bad choices I made. I have to look back. I happen to believe that the things that happened to me don't define me. I believe the things that happened to me or the things I chose to do are the things that help navigate me in a new direction. I just got a little off track, a little off target. I'm just getting back to what I was always supposed to be. So that transformation, we need to embrace it.

Q: It's not only the story that is so important, it's about a transformation. You're bringing inspiration, you're showing that you can make it.
I'm not going to rock myself in a corner and hold on to my sick little blanket. It drives me crazy when I

see that, because it's what you're choosing and there's such power in choices every second of every day. It's the set of glasses you're choosing to look through. People have said to me, "I don't even understand how you can just stand here and be smiling." Let me be clear. To get right down to it, I look at what our Lord had to endure. Nobody understood what he had to go through in order for us to find victory. And not just for the moment, but for eternity. That we would be absolutely set free. There's always somebody who's got it worse than you and somebody who's got it better. All my years of counseling and coaching people took me across the river bed. Because now, I don't look at people in their situation and sympathize. When somebody tells me something, and I know exactly how they feel. Guess what? I have an invitation to speak into your life. When we're doing this, nobody's listening. It's going to be an exchange of experiences.

That's what's so beautiful because I could take my story, I could take the ugliness of it, and never share again. It's too sad. It's too much. It's too heavy. But I could be that broken piece of pottery. I want to shine. Think of a beautiful diamond. When you see a diamond, it's just like a rock. It's not until the artist makes the cuts and the light hits it that it becomes beautiful. I feel like that's what our lives are supposed to be, shining like that diamond.

CHAPTER 5:

"Organizing your home to move forward

with Karen Meade

═══════════════════════════════════

ALL RIGHT, WOMEN with vision. I am excited for my next guest, Karen Meade, who is a professional organizer, public speaker, and author. This is a perfect time of the year to talk about organizing. Of course, every time in the year is a good time, but we're at the end of 2019. We're really excited about finishing this decade, rolling into a new decade, and getting ourselves organized. I'm excited to talk to Karen because this is what she does for a living. The great thing is, she has such an interesting story. Let's get into the details and find out about what drew her into this business.

Q: Karen, welcome!
Thank you so much, Tam. Thank you for having me.

Q: Yes. You are originally from Chicago?
Yes, I am.

Q: That's where I went to college. I love Chicago.
Great. Where did you go to school?

Q: I went to DePaul University.
A lovely, great school.

Q: Yes, great school. Then you moved down to Texas in 1991?
I did. I moved to San Antonio to begin my elementary education career right after college.

Q: You have a background in elementary education, and you did that for how many years?
I taught 3rd grade for four years.

Q: So that must have been your calling?
Well actually, that was a problem—when you're 21, you think you're going to save every child in your class each year, and you naively think you're going to save the world. Then, the next thing you know, you've become a workaholic and the janitor starts escorting you to your car on Friday nights at 10:00 PM, saying, *"You're 21. You need to go out. Get out of your classroom and go have*

fun!" In all seriousness, I have always loved teaching, but at that young age, I hadn't learned enough about setting realistic goals and boundaries with myself. That led to some serious burnout and my personal evaluation of a healthier work life work balance for myself.

Q: How many years from then, did you find yourself in personal organizing?
I think if I'm doing the math correctly, it'd be 14 years after teaching that I started my professional organizing business.

Q: What do you think drew you to that?
There are a couple things. Most of it was just wanting to challenge myself and see if an elementary education teacher, who had zero business background, could really run a business. It wasn't so much about the *organizing*. It was more about, *can I do this?* I was going to prove to myself that I could do this. Once I knew that 20% of all new businesses fail in the first year, and 50% of businesses fail in the first five years, I thought, *okay, bring it on.* I am going to beat that statistic.

Q: My mom, my sister, and my husband are neat people. I know that people who are typically organized don't necessarily want to organize for others. Do you feel yourself to be an organized person?
Absolutely!

Q: Do you drive your whole family crazy with, put this in this particular place and have everything organized all the time?
The answer I want to tell you is no, I don't drive them

crazy, but if I'm being honest, I'm sure I continue to drive them crazy. Part of it is being a mom, being a woman, and of course, being an organizer. So it was like the trifecta of doom for them. Poor things!

Q: Then, you took that love of organizing and started working with other people. Can you work with any type of organizing? There are so many different types you can work with. Just business people and busy moms. So, what do you specialize in?

I didn't go out specifically looking to organize for a certain type of person or situation. I just dealt with the different types of clients that came to me. When I started in 2008, organizing wasn't super well-known, and people heard about what I did through the grapevine. Different people with different needs and different types of assistance reached out to me.

I have worked with a lot of moms. I've worked with a good number of senior citizens as well. They are both incredibly gratifying. I have worked with my fair share of hoarders, too.

Q: I bet that's difficult. It's a deeper situation than just making sure everything is orderly. It's going through a different situation. Do you have to work with a psychiatrist or anything like that, or is it just going there and doing what you know?

It's definitely the latter. I don't work with a particular specialist, and I always put that disclaimer out there. I do not have a degree in psychology, rather my degree is in elementary education. This is my 12th year as a professional organizer, and I've learned a lot about people. I can tell a lot from that initial phone call. There are some keywords that people may say, and I can typically tell the situation that I'll be walking into before I even arrive. There are just some clue words that they'll throw out there.

I can usually determine quite a bit once I've stepped foot in their home, and more often than not, I'm right on the money. Regardless, I can quickly adapt to whatever their personality and current situation is. Some people are very upfront and honest, and they'll just say that they're dealing with bipolar disorder. They'll just share that with me, which is helpful. I know exactly which approach I should take going forward. Our success really depends on how forthcoming they are willing to be. The more I know about them, the more I understand where they're coming from.

Q: What do you think drew you in? Everyone is born with a core message they're trying to say and what they're meant to do in this world. They're trying to say that, and because they're trying to do it, they continue to be drawn to certain types of businesses, people, situations, those kinds of things. It's either to help them to make their message clearer or to show them that this is not the right direction. But you have clearly shown that this is where you're supposed to be. You're not only organized, but you're drawn to this kind of business. What do you think it is that you are trying to say, your core message?
I am pretty firm in my belief that it's two things for me—definitely the desire to help and the desire to teach others how to do better for themselves. I am a teacher and a helper at my core. I sometimes joke that

I'm a glutton for punishment. I've been a helper and a teacher my whole life—pretty much since my sister was born. That is who I am in my heart.

Q: That's something. It makes total sense why you would go into elementary school education, then you would go and challenge yourself to help people in a different way.

I was a stay-at-home mom for a decade. I have two incredible sons, and parenting is hard on your best, and easiest day. I get to help moms at whatever point they're at and empower them to do better for themselves and their family. It's really about helping them and teaching them how to do better for themselves, plus reminding them not to be so hard on themselves.

Q: I think you and I have a similar past. I went through some ups and downs in my life, and I believe it was all purposeful so that I could turn back around and help others to side-swipe those things or help them through. I know we were talking, and you had shared a little bit in your application about some of the ups and downs that led you to the business. You feared that when you were around 40, you couldn't do it. Tell me a little bit about that.

I was 38 years old when it was time for me to go back to working outside of the home. I really wanted to try something that I may not have tried as I got older so I challenged myself to start my business before I was 40. I was afraid that after 40, I may not be brave enough to start my business. There have definitely been difficulties in my life and in my childhood, as most everybody can say. However, sometimes it's harder than others, but I really try to dig down deep and figure some things out about myself, and why I tick the way I tick. Because if I understand where I am coming from, I'm in a much better place to meet people where they're at.

Q: Yes. So, you went into the business. Did you have the blessing of your husband? Was he on board with helping you to try your own business?
Sadly, he was not on board.

Q: What do you think was the biggest drawback for him?
He's a great guy. He's been in the fire department for 33 years now. He's not really a risk-taker, and not quite of the entrepreneurial mindset. From me he needed a steady, solid, predictable income. Thankfully, because of his position, I was able to try to make "a go" of my business. We all know you don't make money right away when you're starting something new.

Unfortunately, he couldn't quite get on board with my dream. I believe he wished that I would just go back to teaching, but I knew I had changed. I started teaching when I was 21, which was incredibly young. At 38, I was fearful that I was not the same person, or teacher, that I had been at 21.

My two sons were six and eight when I started my business. I was afraid that if I went back to teaching, I may not have the patience and the bond with them that I had spent a decade building. I didn't want to be less of a teacher either. I was afraid that I just didn't have it in me to be both a great mom and a great teacher.

I have felt my exes disappointment in my decision to try something that I had a true passion for. I longed for his support and a shoulder to lean on. I know he was very discouraged with me but I started my business anyway, despite his feelings. It was one of the reasons for our recent divorce.

Q: He didn't support you, and you are growing to be the person that you are. I get it. I've been there. I was in the same situation. Believe me.
Really?

Q: Yes, girl. We can have a whole conversation about that.
I am feeling the love between you and I so much right now. I don't love it for you or for me, but here we are.

Q: It's a trip because, just like you, I think you explained it eloquently, not a bad guy, right?
No, not at all. He just couldn't seem to get on board with anything that's outside the predictable, traditional, 9-to-5 career. If I look at the past careers I have had, from teaching to my organizing business, and everything in between, I was always working for a small start-up in various fields, which were not predictable, they weren't safe, and they weren't always stable, but that is obviously what I am drawn to. If there's a problem to be solved, count me in.

Q: Right. Never take the easy road. I always take the harder road. That's a born leader and that's something not everyone is born to do.

Yes, I am a leader, and have been since high school.

Q: Wow. You have 10 employees. Good for you!

I built my business up starting in 2008, and by 2012, I had 10 incredibly dedicated, kind, hard working people on my team. If someone were to ask me about the aspect of the job I loved the best about owning my business—it was 100% about the people who worked alongside me. I learned from all of them just as much as they learned from me. I will tell you, Tam, over time, they held their heads a little higher, their eye contact was more direct, and their voice a little more confident. That was the most rewarding part about working alongside each of them—empowering them. It was the absolute best.

Q: Isn't that something? Not only were you helping and teaching people to do better by them, for themselves, in your business, but you were also creating an opportunity for women to do that working for your business?

Yes, correct. I tried my best to do that.

Q: Now, what made you do that? Did you stop the business for a little while?

I did. I worked hard at my business for eight years. I definitely had burnout and as I now know, clients don't ever reach out initially on their best day. They mostly call on their worst, lowest, most stressful or saddest day.

So, eight years passed and all of those clients who are carrying such heavy burdens, well, their burdens landed upon my shoulders as well. And so after eight years, I was very burnt out, as were the ladies working for me. We felt that we weren't able to keep going at the same pace and provide the same caliber of service we were accustomed to providing our clients. We all needed to step back for a while, so we did.

Q: Getting back into it, you got so burnt out. How long were you out?

I was out for exactly three years, and had a 9 to 5 job in a field that I had zero experience in. You and I were talking a little bit beforehand, Tam, about how if something's not hard or challenging, well, let's just say, there's a little bit of masochism there. So I put myself in a situation where I needed to learn about running Phase One and Phase Two clinical trials. I was coming out of an extremely beat-down and stressful time, and I threw myself into this situation where I had no prior knowledge. Probably not the smartest thing, but I thought that if I go take this job, maybe this will help my marriage a little. So it was a little bit of burnout and a last-ditch effort. After three years of intense learning, the company closed.

Q: Oh my goodness.

Then I was divorced and jobless.

Q: It all happens for a reason.

I know. Look at where I am with you today, which is lovely.

Q: Yes. You went right back to where you were sup-posed to be.

There's a little bit of me that has to—sorry—but give the *middle finger* sometimes. I'm going to show you that I could do it, I can do it, and I am doing it.

Q: You are doing it. How long has it been since you got back in?

I have been back for about 15 months.

Q: How is your experience now that you have had business. How are you feeling now?

That is a great question. Of course, hindsight is 20:20, and with age comes wisdom. I started my business at 38 and I just turned 50. I'm feeling better than I was because I know I have more good work to do!

Q: Which is a lovely age.

I'm feeling incredibly empowered. I have to say, it is hard, it is difficult as far as the money being inconsistent. But I do love what I do. I really am making a very big differ-ence in my clients' lives, and I know that for a fact because of some situations and client events that have occurred. Sadly, a client took her life after we got her paperwork, kids' keepsakes and photo albums in order. They spoke about our organizing team at her funeral. That is when you know that you have made a difference.

Q: Wow! Oh my goodness.

Very heavy. There have been a lot of heavy things.

Q: You take on the heavy, you take on the difficult stuff, you're put together that way. We've been talking about this whole time, and you're built to do that. That's who you are.

I'm the eldest of three. My sister, brother, and I are incredibly close. Between the three of us, there is only a five year age difference. We had a very difficult childhood, and I did the best I could. It's just who I am at my core.

Q: So, what is your goal now for 2020 for your business?

That's another great question. Number one, I'd like to launch a new service in the realm of virtual organizing. There are organizers who are doing that, so I just need to get some thoughts together and get some things set in place. But the idea that I could help people anywhere around the world whom I may not normally work with because of the distance between us. Also, people are sometimes embarrassed and ashamed at the condition that they live in. They're not always ready to open up their home to a stranger for fear of judgment. If I can do something virtually with them where they just show me their closet, I can be supportive and establish a great rapport with them. I can reach many more clients this way, and I think that could be really incredible.

Q: I think that's a great idea and that you would do well with that. There are so many different ways you can attack that. Whether you're going after the person who is trying to organize or you're going after the person who created an organization company, there's so many ways.

That's so true. That's a good point. There are a couple of different audiences to capture with virtual organizing, especially for the person who is a DIY'er. Someone who says, *"Okay, I can do this. If someone could give me a checklist, and a shopping list so I can order the four products I need for my master closet reorg, and she'll check in with me four times in the next two weeks."*, well, that's an ideal client right there.

Q: For sure.

That would be one of my goals. Another goal is to build my team back up. We really excelled in our move management services in the past. Having a team of like-minded individuals working together to tackle a client's relocation is an incredible feeling. It takes a creative and dedicated team to pull off our special kind of magic. A true passion of Karen Meade Organizing is unpacking a client in their new home and making sure that from the day they move in, things make sense, and are where they are supposed to be.

Q: Many people need that.

They do. Once you move in, you don't ever really go back and rearrange things. You don't take all of the plates and bowls out of the kitchen cabinets and start over once you've lived there for awhile. I have good intuition, plus common sense on how to set up a home. Our unpacking services are pretty sweet.

Q: I love it. I am so excited about what you're creating, Karen. So many neat people. My housekeeper came and helped me because I couldn't think without my space being cleaned. It's incredibly important for a lot of people, and I just needed it. I know that what you're doing is God's work, girl.
Thank you, Tam. I appreciate that very much.

Q: Thank you so much, and they can reach you or find you at karenmeade.com. I'll definitely check you out, and I'm excited to keep up with you and look at some ways that we can collaborate.
I would absolutely love that. I can already tell.

Q: Yes, thank you.
Tam, thank you so much. It was lovely. Thank you.

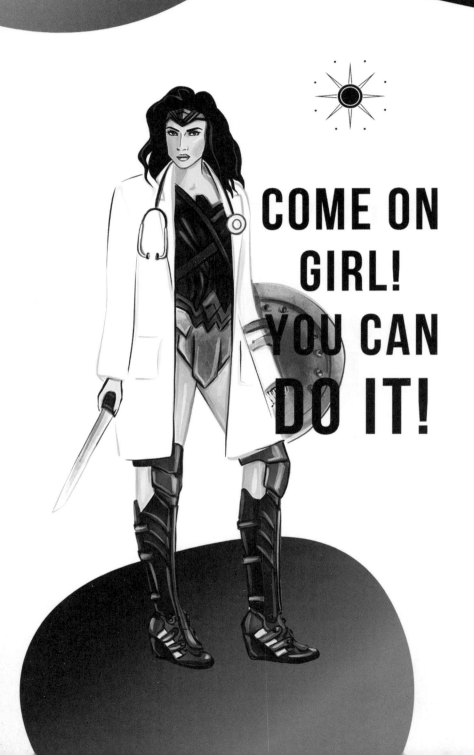

SECTION 3:

Women Who BossUp in Health and Wellness

A big part of the hustle is being mentally prepared. It might not take days or years for you to get going. It could take seconds, but you must click into action. That means being ready when opportunity comes. You cannot count on a job or a company keeping you through sickness and health. With that in mind, it is important to think ahead, take care of your physical and mental fitness, and never give up. I want to introduce you to health coaches and wellness experts who will share their best advice for living well

CHAPTER 6:

"Learning to Cope Without Binging"
with Marisabelle Bonnici

MEET MARISABELLE BONNICI, a pharmacist from Malta. Right now we're in an interesting time because of a worldwide pandemic. As women, entrepreneurs, and moms, we have similar threads. But now, with the world in the throes of Covid-19, we have even more in common. I'm excited to talk about how you are coping during this time.

> **Q: Marisabelle, how are you?**
> Hi, I'm doing well. Thank you. I'm really excited to be here today. How are you?

Q: I am great. How is it going down in Malta? How's everything with you guys?

At the moment, things are heading in the direction of a whole countrywide lockdown. We're in partial lockdown at the moment, so all the non-essential services have been closed off. Officially, it's only food and pharmacies that are still open. And if anybody is caught breaking the lockdown, they are fined or taken to jail. We have several new cases every day. Yesterday, a bus driver was found to be positive. He was driving the bus for a week without a break, which means that we'll probably be seeing a lot of cases coming up.

Q: Oh my, that's too bad. I get it. We've had that same kind of issue here in LA. How are you dealing with that? Are you still working in a pharmacy or has that changed?

I actually owned the pharmacy up to about a year and a half ago. I sold it and we'll probably get more into the reason why later. I'm not working in the pharmacy anymore, which is a good thing because it probably would have driven my OCD a little bit up the wall.

Q: Yes, you're right. Pharmacists are at the frontlines. You have been a pharmacist for a long time. What made you change? Did it have to do with your own personal struggles?

There were two things actually. The one thing that got the ball rolling was the fact that in May of 2008, I consumed some food which was kind of contaminated with rat poison and I was extremely sick and throwing up. I couldn't find a pharmacist to replace me. I owned a very small village pharmacy and our opening hours are set by law. So if we're not given specific permission by the ministry, we're not allowed to close. I couldn't find anyone to replace me even though I was so ill, so I had to keep going to work. At one point, I was literally at work with an IV attached to my arm. I would check into the hospital at night and go back to work in the morning. When I got better after all of that, I decided this is not the life I want to live. I want to live my life. It's not just about the work. Even though I loved my patients and I loved my business, it was not the life I wanted to live. After that, I got that ball rolling in my mind; I started thinking about it. I started realizing that whenever some stress was popping up at work, I was turning to food and binging.

Q: So you were noticing that throughout the years of being a pharmacist, the way you were dealing with stress was with food. Isn't it interesting that the thing that made you stop had something to do with food also?

Yes. It wasn't good.

Q: It was literally killing you. I know rat poison isn't common in food. How did that happen?

There was an investigation because there were a couple of other people who got the same poisoning and apparently it's used in fields. It was spinach that was contaminated. There is apparently a certain amount of time that has to go by before the item can be harvested. In this case, it maybe was harvested before time. That was the conclusion.

Q: Wow. I'm glad to see that you made a recovery and you've made a change in your life and got a chance to start reflecting on your own life and your own struggles. Let's go way back. I know you said you started to see the pattern happening through the stress as a pharmacist, but does it go back even further than that?
I think I can trace it back to my teenage years. I was always bigger than most of the other girls. I'm quite a tall girl. Because of that, I was bullied at school. I looked 10 years older because I was much bigger and developed much earlier. I wasn't fat, I was just a bigger girl. The bullying I used to get because of that used to drive me home to find comfort in food, always. I always loved food. It always made me feel good. So going to school made me feel bad. Being home next to the food made me feel good, and it became a habit. I turned to food every time I was sad, every time I was stressed, and every time I was angry. And that's when it started. I never realized, though, that it was an issue. Even though I was a pharmacist and healthcare worker, I never really realized that I was using food for comfort. For me, it was just part of me. Part of my story. I couldn't see myself without the struggle with food.

Q: It became who you were and how you dealt with life. You know what's interesting? We do things thinking it's working until it's not working any longer. To fill a void, if only momentarily. When did it stop working?
I think I was with my head in the sand for a long time. Whenever someone would point something out with regards to my weight, I would get offended and I would

just say I'm doing fine. Just leave me alone. And I would walk away. It was a Thursday afternoon—I remember, because it was always the quietest afternoon at the pharmacy every week. A guy walked into the pharmacy and we talked. Pharmacists, we do quite a bit of hands-on work. We check patients' blood pressure, their sugars and cholesterol. This patient, a young man, came in and asked me if I would check his blood pressure, his glucose, and his cholesterol. And they were all high.

So, obviously, as a healthcare worker and a pharmacist, I was giving him advice about how to do some lifestyle modifications so he wouldn't need to take medication. I advised him on what he should be eating and how to exercise. He just said yes. And he was very polite. But the look in his eyes was sort of petty, like he was telling me, *Why aren't you doing the same thing yourself?* And it was the eve of a public holiday. I remember I went home and I used to do quite a bit of volunteer work with a woman's association. And the head of this association came to talk to me in the evening about a young girl who needed the HPV vaccine, but she couldn't afford it, and we wanted to find a way to give it to her. After some chats, she asked me how I was doing and I told her that I was okay. But I realized today that I took care of everyone else but I'd never taken care of myself.

Q: I want to just highlight that because that's a struggle for many women. Taking care of everyone else. But why did you realize then? Was it because of that exchange with this guy?
Yes, I think so. That's what triggered it. My friends had been telling me this for ages: *Stop taking care of us and*

take care of you. You're taking care of your family before you take care of yourself. But I never listened. I don't think I've ever met this guy again. It was the first and only time I saw him, but it just triggered something and I kept on thinking about it the following day. I was home all day because it wasn't a working day, and I kept thinking and thinking and I messaged my friends and I told them, "I need your support because starting tomorrow I'm going on a diet." And that's how it started really.

Q: Is this the first time you went on a diet that way?
When it started out, it was just another diet, to be honest. I was really motivated to make it work because I was on the scales. I hadn't been on the scales in two years and I was shocked. I was 150 kilos; I think that's around 330 pounds. And I was thinking, *I can't. If I want to keep doing this, I'm gonna end up in a grave, very soon.* I started doing well. Over the first couple of months, I lost 18 kilos really easily. Then something happened. I don't remember what it was, but I remember coming home and putting everything I could find in the kitchen into my mouth. I was full and I kept on eating and eating and eating.

Then the following day, I remember feeling bad and asking myself how it happened. I asked myself, *Why can't I stop eating?* And I Googled it. Binge eating disorder came up on my screen and I started reading about it and it hit me like a ton of bricks. This is what I do. Something happens, a switch gets turned off. I'm on autopilot and I'm literally stuffing my face with food even though I'm not hungry anymore, just to numb myself out with food.

Q: I think that a lot of us can relate on some level. So then what was the next step for you?

It took awhile for me to actually get to where I am today. I started working out because I thought maybe having that would help my mindset. It did for a little bit, and then it didn't. And the binging started again. Then I started speaking to a psychologist and it was helpful up to a certain extent, but I was still not seeing the results I wanted to see and it wasn't okay for me. I'm a perfectionist, so if I find out something I want to get to the roots of it.

Q: It's been about a year and a half since you stopped your pharmacy. But when you had this big epiphany, how many years ago was this?

2017. It wasn't that long ago.

Q: About three years ago, before you had the rat poisoning in the food. So the first epiphany came with the conversation with this guy. But you still hadn't come to this rat poisoning incident?

Before the rat poisoning thing, I was doing very well. I was reading the research about the mind and how binging works, how the survival parts of our brain are triggered and that is what causes binging. I started learning and the more I started learning, the more I understood and the more I could not beat myself up when something went wrong and I overate, for example. And I'd just move on the following day because it'd started happening less frequently. Then, when the rat poisoning happened, I was not allowed to eat any solid foods for over a month. So I remember my mom used to come over and help me with the food because I couldn't. I didn't even have the energy to cook. And she would make these broths with chicken and then remove all the chicken and I would just have the liquid.

After I started eating again, the binging sort of got triggered again, I think because my body was deprived of food for a long time. And then, once again, my mind wanted to eat again. But you know, now that I knew what the issue was, I wasn't going to let it go. So I kept looking, I kept researching. I started working with a coach who was an expert in the field and I started reading books and doing courses myself. I think it's one of the best things that could have happened to me. Honestly, the whole thing led me to understand and learn more about the brain, more about eating disorders, and it got me where I am today.

Q: Oh my goodness. So where are you today? What is your expertise and what do you help people with?
Yes. Road to Belle started way before this. Way before I even decided to start losing weight in the first place. It wasn't called Road to Belle. It was a blog. It was called Hot Pursuits and it was created for my best friend who wanted to start a website but didn't know how. So I told her, "I'll figure it out." I went online, I went on YouTube, and I figured it out. I created this for her and she just didn't take it anywhere. I went through all the trouble to learn how to do this, I'm not going to let it just stay there. So I started writing about health because that's one thing I knew my patients were interested in and they were taking care of their health better. And when I started to lose weight, I started to talk about my weight

loss journey. Then I said to myself, *I need to change the name of the website. It doesn't quite sound like me.* I'm not into fashion much. I was using this hashtag in Maltese, it's Road to Mazza, which means literally "road to sexy." All of my friends told me that I should change the name of my website to Road to Mazza. And I said no.

Then I thought, Road to Beautiful, because I want to feel as beautiful outside as I feel inside. It's a play on my name as well, since Belle of Marisabelle means "beautiful."

Q: When I first thought about it, your name is Marisabelle so Road to Myself makes sense. Road to finding yourself and getting who you truly are. But Belle means beautiful. I love that. What do you think your biggest hurdle has been?

I think I was my own biggest hurdle, my own mindset. The fact that for a long time I looked in the mirror and I used to see a monster. I used to feel that I didn't deserve to be loved, I didn't deserve to feel good. I just didn't deserve it. So I wanted to give more of myself to help others because I wasn't worthy of it.

Q: It seems as though you were finding your way, working on your mindset, and that started the whole thing. And then you were primed for that conversation to happen, because you were already working on your mindset. Whatever he did triggered something, so you really started to do that work. Then the rat poison incident. It seems there's a reason for everything that happened.

I believe that as well today. I know that there's always

a reason for something to happen. There's always something coming next. Even if you look at the situation today with the coronavirus pandemic, we are all stuck inside. But the earth, the world, is breathing. Who would have thought there would be dolphins in Venice? I don't know if you've been to Venice before, but the waters there were so dirty and stinky and now there are dolphins and swans there. Pollution here in Malta has decreased by 70%.

Q: Isn't that something? It's like the world, the earth, is getting healed in some way. So you were diagnosed with celiac disease about eight months ago. I know a lot of people have gut issues. How is that, to be ethnically Italian and have celiac issues? Everything is wheat, pasta, and bread.

I have to admit that for a while I didn't want to accept it. I was ignoring it. Which, of course, is very bad. I should know, since I am a pharmacist. But I was thinking, *It took me so long to get here, to get over this and be able to have a good relationship now with my food. I'm not binging, I'm not overeating. I'm actually enjoying what I eat without any restrictions or doing strict crazy cabbage soup diets or any other diet that I've done. And now I'm back to having this struggle with my food.* And it took a while. And when I finally accepted that, I started to eat what makes my body feel good. If this food with gluten makes my body feel so bad, I bloat, I am in pain physically, then it's not good for me. I don't want it in my body. I don't want it next to me. It did cause me to put on some weight unfortunately, because obviously my body wasn't absorbing food for a long time. That's what happens to the intestines when they're exposed to gluten for a long time. The weight gain also damaged my mindset a little bit. Because when you see yourself getting bigger and your clothes aren't fitting, you feel negative. But I decided that this is not going to hold me back. I'm actually going to be using this as a learning experience. I can help others who are going through the same situation. The fact is that now my body feels good and I can work out as long as I want. Before, I was working out for 10 minutes and had to run quickly to the bathroom.

Q: Sounds similar to my symptoms.
Yes. My boyfriend is an agriculture specialist and he was explaining to me that wheat has been hybridized so much that now it contains over 50,000 times more gluten than it did 20 years ago. This is why there are so many intolerances being diagnosed and why so many people are having issues with gluten nowadays.

Q: That makes sense. What advice would you give to other people who may be struggling with this particular disorder or something similar, or anything that's really causing people not to be and feel their best?
If we're talking about a binge eating disorder specifically, I want them to know that, first of all, they are not alone. All of our brains work in exactly the same way. We all have this particular part of our brain, the reptilian part of our brain, which controls our breathing, our eating, and our reproduction. If that part is triggered, then that is what is causing us to binge. That is what's causing us to overeat. All they need to do—and it's not as simple

as one, two, three—is stop with the restrictions, enjoy food, listen to their body, listen to how their body feels. How do you feel when you eat certain foods? Are you tired? Are you hungry? Are you full of energy? And start focusing on the nourishment of the food. Forget about the calories. Forget about everything else. Just focus on how your body feels. And once you start focusing on that, you can actually start loving your body as well even more. Then, once you start loving yourself, you'll probably not be binging anymore.

Q: That makes sense. Let's make a little pivot, because we've been talking specifically about binge eating and your personal journey with binging. I want to talk about you making that decision a year and a half ago to walk away from a pharmacy career and start your coaching business. You already owned a business, but completely changed to what you're doing now. What was the reason?

I wanted to live. I just wanted to experience my life. My life at that point was going to work at seven o'clock in the morning, coming home at eight o'clock in the evening to an empty home, because I was only focused on my work so I didn't even have a relationship. I lived alone with my cats and I continued working to 11 o'clock at night. I went to bed and I did the same thing over and over again. And at that point, I decided this is not what I want. Life is short. And I want to enjoy my life. I want to love my life. So, to be honest, it was not that hard of a decision. Even though a lot of people think it was hard. It was not.

Q: So what was the first thing you thought you were going to do?

I didn't know at the time. I had no idea.

Q: I love that answer. And the reason I love that answer is because it really didn't matter. It was going to happen because you were done. What did you do first?

The first thing I did was travel, to be honest. I went to 10 different countries and I just enjoyed being abroad. I traveled with friends. I traveled alone. I traveled with my mother and it was great. It was fun. Then a friend of mine who was pregnant and had to give birth earlier for medical reasons needed me to replace her for a few weeks at her pharmacy. So I did that for a few weeks and I realized what a smart decision it was to leave the pharmacy.

People had been getting in touch with me for a long time to help them with their weight. And I used to just motivate more than anything else because I didn't feel that I was qualified to help them. I used to give advice about nutrients, about how to curb cravings, and about how to keep mentally motivated. And then a friend of mine told me, "Why don't you look into doing this for a living? You love it, you're good at it. People look at you and they can see their journey. You're relatable." And I started looking into it. I started studying more. I did a coaching course. I started reading a ton of books about neuroplasticity and rewiring the brain and I took courses on learning how to reach our goals and all of that. Then I started working with a few clients and helping them reach their goals with regards to loving their body and loving themselves and having a better relationship with food overall.

Q: That's great. Are you much happier with your life now?

It was the best decision in the world. I have an amazing boyfriend whom I love. I can explore things like my photography, which I never had time for. I actually won Photographer of the Year in Malta last year, which I'd never had time for before. I'm traveling, which I've always loved, and I hadn't been doing that since I had the pharmacy. I have faith that my life is going to take me where I want it to take me because I have the knowledge. I have the healthcare knowledge, which also helps when dealing with health issues. I tend to pick things up a little bit more because of my clinical expertise. I know that when you put good vibes out there, the world is going to bring good things back to you. I'm confident of this.

Q: You really represent what it means to boss up. You bossed up for your life, for your health, for your sanity. You bossed up, and it didn't really matter what you were going to do because what was important to you was your life. I love that. What advice would you give to another female entrepreneur who finds herself in a similar situation?

Don't be afraid of your dreams. If you have a big dream, go for it. Write it down on a piece of paper. Keep it in your wallet and look at it every day and start living like you are that person every single day.

Q: Marisabelle, I couldn't have said that better. You are amazing. I'm so glad that I met you and I cannot wait to keep doing things with you. I love being around women like you who are just so clear about their vision.

Thank you. It was a great opportunity.

"You've always
had the power."

—LAUREN D'ANGELO

CHAPTER 7:

"*Yoga and mindfulness*"
with Lauren D'Angelo

I AM REALLY excited today to be talking to my next guest. Her name is Lauren D'Angelo. She's calling us from outside of Boston, Massachusetts.

> **Q: How are you doing?**
> Good. It's always nice when you can start your day with some sort of activity when you feel motivated enough to do it. Especially on a Friday, right?

Q: Especially on a Friday. You're also a fellow writer, so you have a blog and you do some copywriting work. I'm excited to find out a little bit about your journey and how you got to starting your business, Lola Yoga.

Yeah. I've been teaching yoga now for over 10 years. It flew by in a flash. I think before COVID-19, I was up to seven classes a week. Since then it's slowed a little bit as I have been currently teaching online. I got into yoga through running. I was training for my first marathon with my best friend from college. I've been active my whole life and actually started running in college when I had insomnia. So when she asked me to run with her, I said, "Yeah, okay. Sure, I'll try."

So we started training. She was living in New York at the time; I was living here in Boston. She was training in New York; I was training here in Boston. And every Saturday after a long run, when we got on the phone, we would talk about how it went.

Anyway, after I ran the Boston Marathon, I needed something different. Another one of my very good friends brought me to my very first yoga class, and it was as I always describe it - like lightning in a bottle. I knew right away, that second, and there were definitely other things happening in my life at the time.

While I was in corporate America, I was young and only in my 20s. It was really fast paced, I had just gone through a pretty bad breakup, and was wavering and floundering slightly. I had a really solid job, and I loved it, but I wasn't really sure where it was going, not to mention, where the relationship was going. Yoga came into my life right when it was supposed to.

The copywriting and marketing consulting came later. I had to take the leap out of corporate America first, build my teaching schedule and then the universe conspired to deliver my other purpose, again, right on time.

Q: There are many aspects of yoga culture. Vegan, holistic, to hip-hop yoga. Where would you say you fall in that spectrum?

Oh, I am kind of along the whole spectrum, to be honest. I'm open to it all, and I've tried it all. I was a vegetarian for a time, and a vegan for a time. It's part of the journey. In order to know what you like and what works for you, you have to know what doesn't. This practice of yoga accepts everybody.

Even though in recent years there's been this kind of thought on what type of person practices yoga—white females wearing yoga pants—it is a misconception. Yoga began as a form of stretching in order to sit in meditation longer.

It is more than just the yoga poses, it is a way of life. It is a practice of creating a deeper, more meaningful connection with yourself. Many consider the physical practice a moving meditation. When you really take a look at what mindfulness does, it is like holding a mirror up for yourself so you can ask yourself, "how are you being with what you are doing?"

So to your original question. I've tried all facets of this practice. What I've really fallen in love with is the mindfulness that I try to put behind what it is that I'm doing.

If I am practicing asana that day, how do I feel? And if I'm tired, I'm not going to do vigorous practice;

I'm going to do more slow flow and deep stretching, or I'll spend more time in the final pose that everybody loves of Savasana.

When I am off my mat, I practice mindfulness in other ways. It is about myself and self-care, but it is also about my interactions with others. I might consider how my reactions and interactions are with others, what my intentions are for my actions, and checking myself against my values on a daily basis. You could consider this practice or way of life, a practice in accountability.

Q: Yeah. It's interesting, because I love what you say about mindfulness. Yoga is a physical exercise, but it's really more than that.

Oh, so much more. You know, I remember one of my very first teachers that I ever went to. He often would use the phrase, *Just watch. There's nothing to do, just watch.*

And for a long time I was, like, "what is he talking about?" Eventually I came to really understand that so much of this practice is being an inner witness and taking a step back and observing and watching what it is that's happening within you so that you can understand how you're coming across outwardly.

So, much of the work is internal, and much of the internal work requires a lot of listening. So that way you're truly ensuring that you're being your authentic self, and you're on the path that you want to be, and you're also holding space and empathy for yourself knowing that at any moment you can completely start again.

You can wake up tomorrow and be, like, "You know what? COVID-19 has opened my eyes and I'm seeing the universe completely different than I did prior to it." Then, it is about what you are going to do with that. Will you ignore it? Stuff it down? Or welcome the feelings so you can dig deeper and understand what changes specifically you want to see in your life.

Q: Yes. I love that. It's a practice—not even the teacher's practice, it is your own practice.

I'm just a guide. When I step into a room and I'm teaching asana, my job is just to hold space. That's it! And my hope is that the environment I create breaks down barriers, both internally and externally.

Q: What do you think about yoga that appealed to you so much at that moment? When you think back on your life when you were younger, what do you think was prompting you years ago to know this was going to be your road?

I have two older brothers and a younger sister. Both my older brothers, they played soccer. I was on the field next to them playing field hockey through high school. And then my little sister actually followed in my footsteps. This was awesome because she played on the same field and played the same position that I did.

Growing up was rooted activity and movement.. We're all very active, and believe in working hard. My dad owned his own business growing up, and I watched him grow that business to be very successful, and it really inspired me.

I wanted that drive, and I am grateful that I got it from him and my mom. Both parents taught us that hard work is going to get you to where it is that you want to go.

I didn't know that yoga was going to be such a big

part of my life until the universe sent it to me. I was working very hard and struggling with self-care and mental clarity, and then it showed up.

Yoga is like my True North. Where I can check in with myself and really know, okay, how is it really that you're doing?

The asana practice is what lead me to yoga, but the shift into meditation and mindfulness that came along with it was an unexpected surprise and what kept me going back.

Q: What would you say to someone who is feeling like they need that? They need something that's going to help them to start doing that for themselves? Taking time with themselves, checking in for themselves? What would you say is their first step?

Start small, and just keep showing up for yourself. When I first started the asana practice, the physical practice, I struggled to get through a class. My mind was racing, I wanted to give up, I couldn't understand what was happening. But through the movement and connection with my breath, over time, the chaos that was happening during the practice started to let up.

Being patient and knowing that we call it a practice for a reason, and we call all of it a practice, even the mindfulness part. Trust the journey, just keep showing up.

A few years ago, I struggled with anxiety and panic attacks and pretty severe depression. It was circumstances in my life that had led me down that path. Through that time, my meditation practice was nonexistent. I had to learn to start over. I had to learn to be able to sit. When you have severe anxiety and panic disorder, it is so difficult sometimes to just get quiet and sit still.

But just like building a brick house one brick at a time, I had to build my ability to sit with my thoughts, one minute at a time. Eventually, I craved it, and I found myself sitting in silence for 45 minutes a day. But it takes time, consistency, and patience.

Q: What do you think that did for you?

It's completely changed the trajectory of my life. I am clear on who it is that I am. I am more authentic to myself. I'm able to know when to say yes, and when to say no.

Through the process of learning how to manage anxiety and panic, I learned that self-doubt often is created by a story that we tell ourselves and not always rooted in reality.

I often found myself riddled with worry about what others wanted from me, and I was missing what I wanted and needed for myself. This feeling is a common one for us all.

Now, I try to base my actions on what I want and what will bring me the greatest amount of harmony and peace and contentment in my own life.

Q: Right. I love that. You actually started your yoga practice. Would you say you went into business at that time, or do you say that that came much later?

Much later. When I started my practice, I knew right away. Like I said, lightning in a bottle, love at first posture, if you will. I think I left that class that day, I went home, then I signed up for teacher training.

The journey of my teacher training was lengthy.

There was some time in there that I took just to really focus on my practice. And then shortly after that time, I did open a yoga studio. That was a learning experience for me. I realized that it wasn't the right fit. Yoga studio owners have a special place in my heart because it is definitely a business that is not easy. I think the greatest challenge was staying centrally located in one place.

I tend to be a little bit more of a free spirit and want to connect people and know people as much as I possibly can, versus this idea of being committed to that one space, which, by all means, yoga studios owners have the absolute right to do that. I've watched, and I know many yoga studio owners. It is like their first baby, and they really nurture it and they take care of it. I have such respect, and I'm so humbled by them.

So, I did that for a few years. I knew it wasn't the right fit for me. My corporate job took me out to the West Coast for a year, my yoga practice grew exponentially by moving across the country and practicing in California for a year.

Q: Really?

Yes, absolutely. It was just a different location, a different space, a different mindset. I learned so much, and when I was ready and able to come back to the East Coast, I was incredibly grateful to be welcomed back with open arms by the yoga community.

When I moved back I knew that I wanted to be a connector and wanted to be in the community and able to work not only with studio owners and through different studios, but with practitioners. So that is how Lola Yoga was founded.

It is a brand that I created that is the platform to be able to market not just where I teach, but my writings, my podcast, and some other plans I have for the future that are yet to come.

Q: I notice you have said that your intention for Lola Yoga is to be a resource?

Yeah, a resource. While I was having a hard time a few years back, I revisited my love of writing. It's funny, I remember I had an English teacher, her name was Ms. Hoff. It was in fifth grade, and I remember the last day of school she wrote in my yearbook to never stop being a deep thinker and never stop writing. It's amazing what you learn from your teachers and what you take.

When I found my way back to writing, I was amazed at how stuff would just start to flow out of me to the point where I sometimes couldn't stop it and I couldn't get my pencil to move fast enough. It took me a little while to actually be daring enough to put it out there. I kind of dipped my toe, and then I would send it to some friends and ask what they think about it.

But after about a year doing it, Lola Yoga was born. The podcast was a goal that started a year later. The podcasts took me a lot of courage to put it together and have the guts to put it out there.

Q: What are your biggest obstacles that you've had to overcome?

Definitely, failure. It isn't the best feeling when it happens, but I'm grateful to say that at this point I've had enough failure in my life that I look for the lessons from it every single time. I have learned to take it a little bit more in stride, whereas I used to take it so much to heart, it would stop me from progressing on to the next thing. I would like to stew and really marinate and get fixated. I trust more now that from, ruin amazing, things are born. It is a gift that is often missed because we aren't comfortable being in it.

In fact, I hesitate to even call them "failures." Our failures truly are our greatest lessons. Failure is going to happen. So, if we can accept it, and allow it to happen, with a little more loosening of the fear and shame around it, I believe we can all better see what is really meant for us.

I've made many mistakes and I know I am not done making them, but I am not afraid of them anymore. Each time I have made a mistake, I've gotten closer to finding who I am.

Q: Yeah, I do know that about myself. I cannot be held down. We cannot own anything that's like a building. I'll own a building and rent it out as long as I don't have to be there every day.
Right, right. The other thing that I would say is to get clear on what and why it is that you're doing it, right?

Q: Oh yes, girl. Yes. Literally, my whole brand. First, you gotta get clear, you have to nail your message. Why are you doing what you are doing?
Many of my teachers have often challenged me with the "why." In recent years, when I knew Lola Yoga was going to happen, I put pen to paper. My values became more concrete.

Mindfulness, yoga, health and wellness is a crowded

space—so I had to keep going back to my why. I truly believe we are all a work in progress. I am not the holder of yoga. None of us are. I only know the information and knowledge that I have.

But my passion for what I have learned through this practice is something that I want to share so that other people can bloom the way that I have. I don't know if I would be where I am today if I didn't find this practice. I don't think I would be.

I've been humbled by the experiences I have had as a teacher. Students that I have met who have come into my class, and they keep coming. They don't say a lot. They just walk in, week after week. After some time, they'll come up to me and explain that they found their way into the practice because they were experiencing severe depression, or anxiety or going through a bad break-up. Or maybe it is that they lost their job, or a parent, or a loved one. When you hear stuff like that, there is a sense of purpose that you feel. It's much bigger than me. I didn't invent this practice. I just get to communicate it. I just get to be the vessel that it comes through.

Q: What's interesting about that story, Lauren, is that when you came into yoga, you were without direction. You were going through a transition in your life. You were trying to figure out what's going on. You have yoga, and it gives you direction. Your song is also speaking to their hearts and giving them direction. So that's very interesting. Beautiful.

It is. I think I've also learned that through yoga there's also a fundamental accountability that we all have to ensure we are checking in with ourselves on. If we want a different life, then we have to create a different mindset and a different behavior and not get caught up in the stories that create the suffering.

I have often found those stories for me, hold me back. Yoga and mindfulness was the mechanism that allowed me to set the story free and move one from in.

Q: I love it. How do you stay motivated?
I keep going back to my purpose. I keep going back to my "why." I know that this is my passion and my purpose—my dharma.

It's also how I was raised.. My whole family operates this way, in that if you want something, it's not going to be handed to you. If it is handed to you, you probably won't feel a fraction of as good as it would feel as if you worked for it. I had a chance to watch my dad do it growing up, and my mom was a large part of that while she really was raising us, the four kids. We all really watched both of them work very hard, and it flowed through. It keeps me motivated.

Q: Yeah. Well, I love what you're doing. Definitely want to invite people to check out Lolayoga.com. You say you also are teaching online as well. You have an online class?
Yes, I have. Right now, I'm offering online classes. I also offer private yoga teaching, they can also be done virtually.

Q: We'll definitely check out lolayoga.com. I'm excited to be doing this big project and to have you as one of the contributing authors of Women Who BossUp. Lauren, thank you so much, and continue doing what you're doing.

Thank you so much, Tam. It's been such a pleasure, and I'm super excited to be part of this book.

Q: Yes. Thank you.

CHAPTER 8:

"Stay healthy, reduce weight and improve immunity"

with Dr. Usha Mantha

═══════════════════════════════════════

HEY THERE, SUPERWOMEN. I am really excited today to be talking to one of my girlfriends. I met her a couple of months ago. Her name is Dr. Usha Mantha. She is board certified in family medicine and a diplomate in obesity medicine. She is also the founder and CEO of Verve Weight Loss and Laser Aesthetics in Upland, California.

Q: Dr. Mantha, how are you?

I am very well. Thank you, my dear.

Q: I'm so excited. You've helped me a lot. You're an expert in obesity medicine, and you helped me get back on my weight-loss journey. So far, I have lost eight pounds and I feel really great. First of all, how did you end up starting your Laser Spa in Upland? What prompted that?

A little background: Even as a child, as a girl—a little female child—I always looked *up*, for some reason. If my mother gave me a string of beads, I made it into pearls. If somebody gave me a string of laces, I tied it around my ankles. We couldn't afford fancy shoes that tied up, but I had this notion that if you tie up on the ankle and wear some shoes, it just looks more classy and "higher" than what I was.

So I already had this thing going from very early childhood, and gradually it added up with my passion for working with women, with my background of training, and it slowly happened. Then when I was doing primary care, I came across weight management. I was really frustrated, distraught with what overweight and obesity does to patients or clients. And especially for women, how the body changes through childhood to peri-menopause and menopause. For women, it's so much more dramatic that I had to open my weight-loss center.

So, that's where I got my diplomate in obesity medicine. Subsequently, one of my best friends came into my office, and she was really distraught. Her husband, whom she was married to for twenty-five years, walked away with another woman just because she was prettier. Until that time, I worked with women—I see about seven, eight women a day and I talk to about ten women a day—and I had not realized how women were perceived. What was it all about? She said, "You always wanted me to be healthy from inside, but what about my outer beauty? You should have done this, this, this, so I could look pretty." She was in her late forties, the same age as I was at that time. So, I thought, "Oh my gosh, this is what I need to do. This is my calling. I need to make women beautiful from outside while I make them healthy from inside."

Q: Yes. I love that concept.
That's where I opened my Verve Med Spa, or Verve Weight Loss and Aesthetic Center. "Verve" means spirit. Good spirit. Vigor. Enthusiasm.

Q: Oh, I love it. Enthusiasm. If you're in Southern California—you have to go to her spa. It's beautiful. I went there a couple months ago, and it's really well done. But you weren't originally in obesity medicine. You were originally doing what?
I'm very grateful to God. He cultivated me from the get-go for all the things that have come later in life. When I was a little girl, I was so "adjusting" in nature. I had a lot of resilience. I was like that from a young age, and of course, I became a medical student. After that, I went straight to London.

So, in England, I spent ten years in Obstetrics and Gynecology, and that's where my love affair with women started. I make this joke that I am one of those who spent a good eight to ten years between women's legs, because I feel like I have the entitlement to say so. I'm entitled to say so. I have been passionate for women's health. Every single woman who touches my life, I want to improve her life if I can. If I am allowed. So, that's where I'm coming from. I did my training in OB-GYN in England, and subsequently, I went to Pennsylvania. That was about twenty-four years ago. At the time, I switched to family medicine because it gave me a broader platform to help more people. And women are called for their family. I wanted to be closer to women and their families. So, I became a family physician. I've got twenty years almost of being a Board-Certified Family Physician. That is when I realized how important it was to train in obesity medicine. Remember this, Tam, obesity medicine, anything to do with weight management, is not taught in medical schools.

Q: I didn't know that.

We don't have time for learning how to manage being overweight. We read all about what it can do to the body—high blood pressure, cholesterol, sugar problems—but we don't have a curriculum for anything to do with weight management. We assume we know about it. It's not that simple. When your body changes before and after childbirth, you think, "Oh my gosh, what happened?" And most of us women are so busy between ages twenty-five and forty-five in our lives. Twenty years of our life is gone in childbearing, child rearing, and childcare. So once children are out of our house when we're forty-five and fifty years of age, now we are slammed with peri-menopause. In fact, last night I was in another women's group talking about menopause. It was a blast because everybody's like, "Is this what happens with us? Nobody told us this."

Q: Nobody tells us this. I know. It's so true.
We are just thrown from one type of life to another life to another life. I mean, when the periods come, we have no idea. We are shocked. Everybody's like, "Shh." Especially cultures back in India—you know and I know, we come from other countries—how much is taboo to grow up. Whereas, it's our physiology. So, seeing all these things about women, coming from a family with five sisters, I'm the best person for women's health care. That's kind of where I came from.

Q: I love that you brought this up. You guys are just going to fall in love with Dr. Usha like I have, because her resilience is so apparent in so many different ways. You came from India originally. That's where you were born, and you're the number-four child, right?
Number-four daughter, Tam.

Q: Yes, number-four daughter. And if you don't understand about the culture and how things go, this is really good education to see where her passion even comes from. So, tell me about that. Coming in and your family.
So, coming in, my father was educated; he was an engineer. But back then—we're talking about fifty-five-plus years ago—having a boy, having a male child, was supposed to be the progression of your name, your genes.

Women, the girl children, were only to be brought up to be given away. I was number-four daughter, I was dark, and in India and all these countries outside we're obsessed with whiteness. We want a fair child. I was the number-four daughter, I was plump, I was dark, and those were all against me. So, when I was born in the hospital, my aunt just peaked through the room and said to my parents, "Another daughter?" And she walked away. She didn't even see me.

Of course, I'm very blessed. I have never regretted my birth or my life. I love it. I have three older sisters who embraced me. My mother was busy trying to have another baby. Of course, they still wanted to. Next to me was my brother. So, there, they got lucky. My brother came along within two years of me being born. And then they tried again, of course, had another daughter—which is all blessed, everybody. However, I kept joking with my aunt for a long time. I said, "Do you know, Auntie, that I became a doctor? I can treat you." And she would say, "Yeah, I knew when you were born." I said, "No, you didn't. You actually were mad at my parents." I'm very grateful they created me for God's sake. I wanted to be created. Look at life. I've never given them grief. I have taken care of my father and my mother every single day. And if it's Mother's Day tomorrow, last night, I already spoke to my mother and I gave her kisses.

This is very important, Tam. We don't know why people go through a certain thing. Good, bad, or whatever—I don't know why I met you. Right? You didn't know I existed. But there is a reason. Reason for even fifty-five years ago why it happened. Of course, the person I was, I got into an arranged marriage and I went to England, and that's what life was. But the joke remains between me and my aunt forever. That, remember I was the fourth, dark daughter.

Q: Oh my God, I love that. So, you got into an arranged marriage. You went to London. Your husband was a doctor? Was he going to medical school as well?

He was. He was a doctor and mine was a fairytale marriage. But, you know, in those days, you saw the person for two minutes and you were married. There wasn't dating, you didn't know anything. In my case, I literally lucked out. My husband was Prince Charming: tall, dark, and handsome. I was very blessed because my in-laws really did their homework about me. The only thing I told my father, I said, "Dad, they are all so excited. They're already calling me daughter-in-law, but do they know how tall I am?" Because, Tam, one thing, I'm very blessed again. I went to a nuns' convent school and they always taught me to stand straight. In fact, when you stood with a hunch, they would come and beat your back and say, "Stand up." They said, "You always stand straight." And I somehow really literally took that into my brain.

So, I told my father, "I hope they know how tall I am"—because, Tam, you've seen me, I'm almost six feet tall. I did not want to be rejected because I was tall. I was an educated girl. I did finish my medicine, and I was very proud of that. My father told me, "No, they know that you are so tall." I must say, my husband was amazingly handsome. Then we went to England.

We really struggled, Tam. Marriage is—it doesn't matter whether it's arranged or a love marriage, it's all individual cases. We have to have zero judgment about marriages. Because it was really hard to be married to a man you see for five minutes, then ten minutes, and in two or three months, you're married and you move in with them. It was really a struggle. Very hard. Then we went to England and we struggled for a good two, three, four years in the beginning. Then we got settled. Then we moved to the United States, and of course, life changed yet again.

Q: Yet again. Tell me about that.
After a few years of struggle in England, we got our memberships from the Royal College of Obstetricians and Gynecologists. That's who I am. Training was seven years. We worked very hard. My husband was a member of the Royal College of Physicians, and for some reason, a friend of ours was visiting and he said we need to go to the United States. I said, "No, we don't," and he said, "Yes." So, Tam, just so you know, wherever you plant me, I like to just be there. I don't want changes. I don't like changes. My whole family laughs at me and they're like, "You are the one who's saying you don't like changes. You went to America, you went to England, then to the East Coast, to the West Coast. You don't stop." I'm like, no, I don't like changes. Anyway, it's destiny.

So, he comes home, he says we're moving to Hershey, Pennsylvania. I'm like, no, we're not. He said, "Yes." One good thing is, even if I don't want to, when I do take up a task, Tam, I put everything in. I just decided, God wants me to do this, I'm going to do this. Anyway, we came to Pennsylvania about twenty-four years ago. We became residents again. In England, we had reached the attending level. We could have had a house, we could have had a salary, and we could have started our life properly. I already had one son at the time, but never mind—we started all over again in Pennsylvania. Fourteen years after marriage, and we moved to Western Pennsylvania, where I got my residency because I studied for all my USMLEs [U.S. Medical License Examinations] and stuff. We finally bought our first house after fifteen years. Okay? However, at the time, my husband started having symptoms.

One-and-a-half years into buying the house, he started having hoarseness of voice. He used to teach residents also. He was a neonatologist outside Pittsburgh, Pennsylvania. He used to fly with little babies because he could intubate little tiny twenty-eight-week babies. He was so skilled. And he started having hoarseness of voice. From July to September of 1998 was really life changing for us. On the 22nd of October, 1998, he came home and he said, "Usha, I'm really, really sorry." I said, "Why?" He said, "I have been diagnosed with advanced cancer." So, twenty years later, Tam, I still can't stop crying. Here's a six-feet-tall guy and he's so accomplished and he's a physician, he's a neonatologist, and he says, "Usha, I'm so sorry. We have two children, but I won't be there." I'm like, "No, you will." He had advanced metastatic cancer. He was loaded with lesions. He did have a change in his mental status. He was depressed. I didn't know why.

I have to tell you this, that when you have extensive

metastasis in the brain, it can change your personality. He was a changed man. After struggling side by side, hand in hand, neck and neck for fourteen years to get where we wanted to, within three months, this person was absolutely a guy I didn't know. We were sleeping in different rooms, we were fighting, and he was forgetting. But when I got the diagnosis, I thought, "Oh my God, this is what was going on." He was riddled with metastasis. My whole life changed on that October day because he was given six months to live. Of course, he was religious, and he had very good family support. So, there was a whole different life change. Literally, as if somebody pulls the rug from under your feet. When that happens, it is a situation you will never forget. That was another journey. I think I was reborn at that point. It was a rebirth for me. I literally changed from being a young, yuppie, careless physician and go-getter, like, I don't care, I will make money, and I'll do this and I'll do that. All of a sudden, I actually became a different person.

Q: **Yeah. Explain that. Because I know at that point you had two boys, right? You're in Hershey, Pennsylvania. Now, you have to become a caregiver to a man who was in late-stage cancer. So, tell me a little bit about how you became a changed person.**

He was just thirty-nine years old and I was thirty-three or thirty-four. You know, when we talk about other people, when we talk about this, even right now in the middle of a pandemic, we are talking about COVID, it can happen to others—Tam, we have to stay humble. It can happen to us. Because it happened to me, out of a family in which both sides of the family are still there. Everybody, right? I couldn't figure it out. His grandfather lived to ninety, his grandfather lived to one-hundred years old. Why did he come up with this mutation? Why did he develop this advanced cancer? It was really posing some questions in my life. I was still a resident at the time, and I decided overnight that it is not a time to feel sorry for myself. I will never, ever feel sorry for myself. I think when we have everything going for ourselves, Tam, we feel vulnerable. When you really don't have any avenues, guess what you get? You get brave. You get empowered.

Q: Yes. And this is really what I mean by "boss up." This is actually what it really means to me.
The adversity of some unknown dimension. I want to share this with your audience. This kind of pandemic. That was a pandemic of my personal life back then. Now, this pandemic has leveled the grounds for every single person. Male, female, young, old, haves and have nots, black, white, poor, brown, Asian, non-Asian, Caucasian. Doesn't matter who they are here. We are all leveled up, Tam. We are leveled up, for some reason. That's how I was twenty years ago. Just in my own journey.

So, I decided to stop feeling sorry for myself. I read lots of books to get through this. I still had to put my kids onto the bus. I was teaching to become an attending. I was drawing the labs from my husband's body because he had to stop driving the very next day. Very next day, he was bombarded with radiation. He had to get full-body radiation and he couldn't drive ever again. Of course, a year and a half later, he passed away. You know, it really brought out all these things in me that I didn't know I had. I had no idea I was so strong. But I stopped feeling sorry because of what I read somewhere. I said, I wasn't the person you need to be sorry for. The person who left this world was. You need to feel sorry for him. After all, we're here to enjoy the day-to-day things. We are enjoying celebrating with each other. Birthdays, weddings, day-to-day eating, drinking, hanging out, and he's the one who couldn't enjoy anything, and he worked so hard for it. So hard that life seemed very unfair. So, in the beginning, I did feel sorry for myself for a little while, but then I stopped because I had read this, and I thought it made sense. What am I sorry for? I'm still here. For the life insurance I fought for—every time I wrote the amount for his life insurance, I fought with him. I said, "We can't afford this. We can't afford this." And guess what? After twenty years, I get that money to bring my kids up.

So that makes me think, "God had a plan." I didn't see it. He bought a large life insurance, larger than what we could afford at that time. We fought every time, every month. Of course, he kept saying, "I'm going to make some money." And you know what he meant? He will make money after he dies. That is for my kids. Tam, I'm so humbled and I keep thinking, "Oh my gosh, God always has a plan." We just need to see it. We need the plan. Like I said, I became a different person. I went to India for two weeks after he passed away, then came back and started working and never, ever have stopped.

Q: You never stopped. Yeah.

You know why? My work is my solace. When I go, I sit in my office. I diagnose one more cancer. I diagnose one more bad thing. I am just sitting there and thinking, I feel how it changes lives. I feel every step of it.

Q: Yes. Well, you have experienced so many changes in your life—as a woman, as a businesswoman, as an educated woman. You've experienced a lot of different situations, and I think that's all so helpful because you do deal with women and you do understand what they're going through at the different changes in their life, and you are usually at the forefront of change. Big changes.

One thing I realized, change is going to happen all the time. It's inevitable. The more we resist change, the more we get it. Every place I went to work, they wanted to give me a job, and I said, "Okay, I'm settling down here." But my husband was a visionary, and I know what the word "visionary" means, Tam. My husband was sick. In the middle of his chemotherapy, he was filling my forms for California. He kept telling me, "You've got to go to California," Tam. I'm so sorry that I came to California without him, and I'm so blessed I remarried. I'm blessed that I found another person.

So, I can be sorry for what I lost, but I have to be very mindful of what God has given me. You have heard multiple conversations when I have complained. I have bitched with you. Stay the course, Dr. Mantha, stay the course, Usha. It's going to be alright. I think that is what I worked for. I also told you I don't want to lose you as a friend because I'm having these issues.

Because issues will happen. Events will happen. People come and people go. People go, and there's nothing you can do about it. Whether they leave you in person, in spirit or physically, whichever way. Because I lost my husband, I gained California. I resisted moving, I resisted change, and I still came to California. I can't complain, because when people look at me, they're saying, you're complaining for what?

Q: You've done an amazing job. Now, I'm going to do a little switch from personal to business. Once you came to California, you started your business, you started your practice. What has been the biggest hurdle that you've had to overcome since starting your practice and then becoming an entrepreneur?

When I came to California about fourteen years ago, I started working for a group practice. That went okay for the first four or five years, but being a leader in my mind, in my personal life—because I had to lead, I had to take command, I had to boss up against my husband's sickness. I had to be the boss. I had to be a boss when my husband passed away. I had to be a boss in my own career. I had to take the lead, and every time we take a lead, we become a boss. We boss up, because women are not supposed to be bosses. We are supposed to be submissive; we are supposed to take orders. When we have to give orders and wear that bossing-up suit, every time, it transforms you higher and higher. So, I did that continuously.

I moved from the East Coast to the West Coast all by myself with my children. I kept doing these things. When I came to California, I worked with a group and I had this thing in my mind: I need to become a businessperson to run my practice as I want. I think that the only way to live your dream and your passion is to do it your own way. If we don't do it in our own way, then somebody else's way is what we have to do. The more I listen to people who have taken this stance, Tam, the more I get connected. I didn't realize that that's what I was doing, but I'd already been doing that. That's how, about ten years ago, I went into a solo practice. Solo practice was unheard of. I had so much resistance from the group. They didn't like me. They hated me for my guts. They kept telling me to my face, whereas I paid them money. So whenever they said, "Oh, you are a traitor," I said, "No, I paid you money. I work very hard. Stop saying that." And they had to stop saying that. They got mad because I was a good person for them to make money off of, but I had to go into practice for myself. I took the punch. I was blessed because I married my current husband, and he did support me.

So, I'm very grateful for that. Gratitude is one thing I think we have to remain in completely. If we are not grateful, how are we going to be more powerful? In order to get more powerful, we pull ourselves down in gratitude. Gratitude is a positive thing. We're not sucking up to anybody. We're just remaining saying, "I'm so grateful I was given that opportunity." I bought my practice from the company, and I had been in solo practice. Then, about five or six years ago, I really wanted to treat overweight and obesity. I was so passionate, and I'm so blessed, I did tons of courses. My husband said, "Do you really have to do like six courses in a year?" I said yes. I sat through halls, I fell asleep, I took notes, I have tons of papers, I did the exam. It takes eight to ten hours of computerized exam, but I did that too.

Then the life-changing event happened about three years ago, when my friend who came in. At the same time, I had really launched my Verve in a very official manner, with lasers. And that threw me from just being a doctor into a true businessperson. Because now, I have a medical spa. Now I'm really, literally doing things to women to make them look beautiful outside. I'm doing injections, I'm doing Botox and fillers and Kybellas, and women are transforming. So I was saying, three years ago, it really occurred to me, I have embarked on a business. Until then, it was a soft professional business. From then on, it became a real entrepreneurial type of business.

Q: Yes. A real business. So, through your story you've been talking about different things, like gratitude and passion. But I know you have some building principles that you would want to share with any woman who wants to boss up in her own life or her business. What are those?

So, a step before that, may I just go over the hurdle that you asked me about so then I can come back to this point? The way I started my business—I really did not plan. I'm a Type-A personality, I'm a busy bee, if you give me a job, I'll get it done. But in that process, being so hyper super active, I didn't realize what it takes to build a practice or build a business. I did not pay attention to the small details. I did not pay attention to having a business plan. I needed to know how finances will work. I needed to know what personnel you need. What is social media? Who do we talk to? Who do we not talk to? What will my website look like? Because different people will give us different ideas and suggestions, I was very vulnerable and I worked through FOMO, the fear of missing out. So, anybody who came with any ideas, I wanted their help. But it wasn't their fault; it's my fault that I didn't know what the heck I wanted.

My biggest hurdle was that I didn't know how a business starts. I just plunged into it and tried to swim. But I must say, this whole COVID thing has given me more time, more energy, more clarity, and, fortunately, within the last six months, people I have associated with—of course, you are included, Tam. I have seen things more clearly. I am understanding what the process is, and so my hurdle has been not knowing. And then, I think, whenever there is a setback, you lose your own confidence. You have self-doubt, like, "Is this something I should have done this way?" Then there will be somebody who'll say, "You shouldn't have done it this way," and that brings you down. And that brings me to your current question—what is it that keeps us going? What are the blocks of my strength, right?

Number one is integrity. For me, fortunately, it came as a child. My sister tells me she loves me, but she hates me because I couldn't keep any lies down. If she made a mistake, I was the very first one to tell my mom and dad, and she would get the beating and I would not get anything. I never got reprimanded. I came out a winner. She's only two years older than I am, and she's like, "I loved you, but I hated your guts. How did you pull this thing through? You were always after integrity." Then I became blessed by going into medicine and the practice of medicine. A practice of medicine is full of integrity. If patients can't trust me—you don't want to put your life with somebody you don't trust. Today, I must say, I'm very lucky that if I do present a plan to my patients, they will accept it nine out of ten times. The tenth one, if they don't, they know I will get them to the next best thing there is. So, I think integrity in all shapes and forms is absolutely necessary. It is a learned phenomenon, by the way. Somebody else asked me, "If you don't have it, can you learn it?" Of course, you can learn it. You can learn any behavior. So, integrity is important.

The second one is passion, which you have mentioned. You are very supportive of that. Without passion, really, nothing moves. Everything moves because of passion. I said this before, even the counters in Macy's and Bloomingdale's—in the front half of their whole building, they have the maximum revenue in these lipsticks and lotions and potions and eye makeup. Because we are passionate as women, we spend another ten minutes, we buy something that we absolutely didn't need. But that passion—whether it's for stuff, for people, for an art, for mountain climbing, whatever it takes—I think passion drives us. Even if we are angry and upset, we need to bring it back to the passion we like, right? So, that is important.

Resilience. If life keeps knocking you down, you need to get up and say it's okay. Just dust it off and go. It's not easy sometimes. After I lost my husband, after I started the business, many times I've wondered at night, did I do the right thing? Why did I do this? But I wake up in the morning and I bring something else—something else I look at and say, it's worth this thing. So partly it's resilience, partly it's your ability to knock the negatives out of your way and stay positive, keep your motivation in front of you. When the children were little, they were my motivation. I wanted to get them through colleges, and I still say to them, "Now you get married and you're on your own, guys. If you don't choose the right partner, don't come to me." I tell them, if you want mommy to marry you, I can take responsibility. But if you marry on your own, you're on your own, what am I going to do? You can't ask your mother every step of your relationship. So, I feel like that's done.

My next big motivation is that I really want to work with women outside the country with childbirth. Tam, one of my passions is to teach obstetrics. I'm very good at it. I love it. I understand obstetrics very well. I don't practice, but I teach. I'm an advanced life-support trainer and advisory faculty through the American Academy of Family Physicians. I want some time-independence and financial-independence. Both are necessary for me to go away and help these nursing schools and teach basic safety in childbirth. If we can make mothers safe through the process, that is what good development of civilization is, to save the mothers, because there is still very high mortality with childbirth. But young mothers don't have to die. It's just so sad. So, that is my passion, by the way—the real passion. I'm waiting, in a year or so, when I'm free from all these things, I can just do this for fun and then go and work there. So, these are my blocks. My strengths.

Q: I love it. I love everything that you have done throughout your career. I love how your business is developing and the learning process and all the gems that you've shared with us today from that journey. So, Dr. Mantha, I am so happy that we did this, and I am excited to do a bunch of other stuff with you in the future.

Thank you, Tam. I'm grateful for your friendship. You and I have had some nice talks, and I know you are an amazing person. I think one of the other important things is to surround yourself with amazing people, because everybody has a story. We just said that. It's unique to you. Unique to me. Even after talking so many times, we still don't know so much about each other. That's what life is there for.

Q: That's what life is there for. That's right. Well, thank you so much for coming on and I look forward to talking to you more soon.

Thank you.

"Don't live in the past thinking about the mis- takes you made. Learn from them and move on. Make them as your fuel to keep going."

—TAM LUC

CHAPTER 9:

"OWN your Life Without Boundaries"

with Victoria Plekenpol

HEY THERE, SUPER women. I am so excited today to have my next guest. I met this woman about a month ago. I was introduced to her from another kick-butt business owner. First of all, I saw her information on her Facebook page that she was living in Shenzhen, China, and I was like, *This woman is living in China. What's going on?* So, I was so excited to meet her and find out her story.

Q: Victoria, how are you?

I am incredible, because I choose to be, right? It's a choice we all get to make daily.

Q: Her name is Victoria Plekenpol, and I'm so excited to have this conversation. She has an amazing health and wellness business that helps people to not only become healthier, but also find a way to help them with their wealth, help them build their business. You can't be able to build a business without being healthy. They go hand in hand. I love what she has created. She is one of the fastest-growing in this business and has one of the most international teams. I'm just so excited because it's incredible to see a woman doing this, and having her daughter be a part of her business. It's just incredible, Victoria. So tell me what inspired you to start doing that?

Can I take you back in time a bit? It's not like I woke up one day and said, *Gee, I think I'll start building an empire today*. It's been a process, a journey. I want to share that I was just that average American kid. In middle-class America, I grew up kind of eating macaroni and cheese. Am I allowed to say that? Seriously, I was just a "normal" person, whatever that means back in the day. Then I had a really transforming moment—a very unexpected cardiac event in my life. I ended up having heart surgery. It completely blindsided my whole family. It was in that season and in that process—and there's a thousand details around it, but it was in that process where I had my epiphany that life is fragile and it can be gone in a moment. That was one part, but the other part was that I had more control than I thought. I had control, by my diet, my exercise, my thoughts and I had control of my choices. I tell my kids this all the time, *Live your life.* Don't watch somebody else's on TV.

Q: Right.
You know what I'm saying? We are her to live our lives—we have a purpose.

Q: Yes.
I don't wish for a cardiac event on other people, but sometimes I meet people and I think to myself, *You need to have something happen in your life that wakes you up and gets your attention.* So many people are sleeping through their lives—just going through the motions. I was just going through the motions the first 20 years of my life, and then I had this event at 21, and I am so glad I did because it woke me up.

Q: That's what's incredible about your story, Victoria, because you had this epiphany early. Twenty-one years old, this happened to you. I didn't have that jump start, kick start and kick in my butt until I was, like, in my 40s. Amazing, right? And so you decided at that time that you can make a choice.
I raised my kids knowing this because I don't want them to have to either have an event that's difficult or wait until they're 40 or 50 to figure out who they want to be. This is a lot of people's paths because they spend the first half of their life just doing what's expected— the social norm if you will. That being said, if you are reading this and you're in your 40's or 50's - It's never too late to start! I'm raising my kids knowing that life

is a gift and they have a purpose, so let's figure it out. Let's figure out what that purpose is and do it.

Q: And get at it! So, I love that it's never too late. It's also obviously never too early either, right? I think that's what your daughter is getting. It's never too early to get it!

Yes, exactly. Even my 10-year-old. When the pandemic started, we thought, *What could we do to make things better?* And she came up with the idea of "Positivity Rocks,". So, we painted rocks and put positive messages on them. We then went around the neighborhood passing them out. She knows she can make a difference at 10 years old—because I have told her over and over that this is the truth.

Q: Of course she can; we all can if we choose to. So, tell me, what do you think your biggest hurdle has been? Not just in your business, but throughout your life?

That is a huge question. I don't think anybody ever has just one hurdle. If you think about competitive racing, they're jumping several hurdles in the race—such is life! I would say that the first hurdle was my health. The second hurdle was probably when I got married. We started moving internationally, and I don't think I realized that this was going to become our life. I've lived in six countries and had three kids, two cats, and one marriage. It's been challenging, and it's been exciting. It's been good and it's been hard. The hard part is that it makes me feel like I'm in a constant state of grieving because I am either leaving, or my friends are leaving. How do you deal with that? It's not something you are really prepared for. How do you choose to deal with that in a positive way?

There's a lot of negative ways that people deal with that. I have seen depression, alcohol or shopping to fill the void—very difficult and sad. So, I had to choose—intentionally—positive ways. Some days were very lonely and challenging. I started really working out of a calendar and then OBEYING MY CALENDAR! I would schedule in positive, healthy activities—and then when I started my business, I scheduled in success! The next hurdle has been health challenges for my kids that have come up. How do you face those? Sometimes, I would just feel tired and want to pull the covers over my head. I actually did that once. I laid there for about 20 minutes and then I got bored and had to get up! I said, *Okay, I can't do this—I need to figure this out!* So, I tried figuring out what the problems were and how are we going to deal with this, fix this, make this better. Sometimes, I would be in China or Amsterdam or some other country when a health problem hit and trying to figure it was not straightforward for me. Let's just say I learned a lot about having grit.

Q: I love that, because it is challenging for all of us - different things. The added layer for you has been you're a professional expat. You've been in so many countries. How long have you guys been traveling?
Twenty-six years.

Q: Twenty-six years. And you're now living in China, normally?
Normally. I've been kind of evacuated. We got quarantined

and then evacuated and then quarantined again. My husband came back to the States and we were quarantined again! We were open for two weeks and then Colorado went into shut down. *I feel like I'm living a whole lifetime in 2020!!*

Q: I think we all are.
2020 has definitely thrown us a curveball. But again, how are you going to deal with the curveball? We get thrown curveballs in life—all the time. Nobody's immune to them—are you going to figure out how to catch them or just strike out?

Q: What I find so fascinating about your story is how you use all those things as a reason why you CAN. A lot of us have so many excuses. There's so many things that I could pull out of your story and say, This is the reason why I can't. You've been moving around, you've been in all these different countries, and you still have been able to build an empire.
That whole moving around, sometimes makes people think, *Oh, that sounds so glamorous and fun.* It is hard work, people! Try getting an electrician in China when you don't speak the language. Good luck with that!

Q: If nothing else, I think that people should get from reading your story, is that you can do anything as long as you decide that that's what you're going to do! Then get at it!
Everything is figure-outable.

Q: Everything is figure-outable.

It's just making the decision to do it and then getting up and DOING it.

Q: You're in Colorado because of the quarantine— you've been on this roller coaster for a little while.

Currently the borders are shut and we cannot return to China.

Q: Do you have any idea when you guys are going back?

No, I am telling everybody my feet are planted firmly in midair. It's like being in a total free fall right now. I was just sharing with a friend yesterday that it's like I got up and today I live here. So, *What can I do today -from here? What can I do to move my family forward? What can I do today to move my business forward? What can I do today to move my health forward?* All I can really know right now is what's going to happen today. I don't know about tomorrow.

Q: This is where I am right now. I'm here.

This is where I am right now. So, now what?

Q: How do you stay motivated?

I'm sure you've heard this before, but EVERYTHING can be your excuse. Everything can be your excuse not to do something, or your reason why to do it. Again, YOUR choice.

Q: Yeah, that's right.

If you want to stay motivated, which of those should

you focus on? Your bucket of excuses, or your vision board with your *WHY*? I'm telling you, vision boards work, people!! They absolutely help you stay focused on the right things!

Q: They do work. They really do pull you forward.
They do. Your *why* should make you cry, and your *why* should get you out of bed in the morning. Your *why* should be big enough that it makes you pick up the phone and call that person that scares you. If you don't have that *why*, then you really need to go into the process of discovering your purpose. A lot of people I meet have dreams that have died somewhere along the way. We all dreamt when we were little kids. We wanted to be an actress, or a ballerina, or a surgeon, or a fireman. We all had these dreams, and somewhere along our journeys, they just got crushed out of us-buried deep inside - forgotten. And so many people have ended up in this - I like to call it the "beige cube," or you've ended up just going through the motions of every day—but everyday compounded equals your LIFE. We go to college, get a job, get married, have kids, buy a house - because that's what we are told we are supposed to do. Nothing wrong with any of that. I did all that, too. Nothing wrong with it, but it's there—this expected path we are supposed to take. But, there's something within all of us—that dream that's been buried is still there. We're all here for a reason that's bigger. If we are courageous enough to tap into that and if we want to, it can have an impact. The impact we were created to bring.

So, the question was, what motivates me and what got me started? What really motivated me to start my business originally was the products that helped my daughter. My 10-year-old has a blood disorder. When I was introduced to my company, I was so skeptical, but I was desperate enough to try and the products worked—they changed everything for us. My WHY was born then—I needed to tell other parents that there was a way to support their children naturally. My daughter lost her hearing moderately in both ears due to an overdose of antibiotics—she will wear hearing aids for the rest of her life. If I could empower parents to support their kids- and not have this become their story—I was Game ON!

"Whys" morph. They evolve, they develop and they grow and they shift and they change. And sometimes you may have three smaller whys at the same time, and sometimes there's one big WHY. And that's fabulous! But, I encourage you to keep track of them on a vision board. My first motivation was to help my daughter thrive. She was so sick. So, I needed to help her thrive. This gave me purpose. That was my first ah-ha moment - *I can educate all these people and help them.* Then I started making money. Then I was like, *Oh, wait a minute. There is more I can do!*

I've got my big overarching *why* now, and it is to help pay for people's adoptions. This is the impact that I want to have because I've seen the impact of adoption in our family. We gave Kailin a forever home, and yes, she's blessed, but we're even more blessed to have her.

There's this gap between the orphanage and the family called $30,000. There are absolutely gorgeous, amazing people who want a child— they would be incredible, loving parents—and they don't have

$30,000. If I can help bridge that gap, that's my over-arching *why*.

However, there is this other element that happened. I have become addicted to other people's *whys*. I have all the people that I work with, and they go on this journey with me—First, they have the health transformation with the products. Then they start to feel better. They start to have energy. They start to have a clear mind, get rid of the fog, and they start wanting to share this experience with their friends—then they want to build a business so they can have *their* WHY become a reality. Then, it's like helping that little child inside remember the dream. It's so much fun helping them develop their *why's* and then helping them to build their business, being a part of making their dreams come true. It's the most incredible feeling to know that I have the power to help people. Almost like a super power to empower!

Q: The power to change people's lives.
Then there's the ripple effect, because they then go and do the same thing. It's truly incredible.

Q: I do think that's incredible. Now you are continuing to grow your business, no matter where you are. Helping a lot of other people to get healthy and to build their businesses. What do you think is in store for you now? What are you really super excited about?
It's a unique season. Let's call it that. So, it's going to be exciting to see the opportunities that come from this.

Q: To say the least.

Again, with my feet firmly planted in midair, I don't even know where my daughter will be going to school next year, it's a little hard to visualize too far down the road. What I'm thinking about right now and what's happening right now is what I've been calling the Pivot.

Q: Oh yes. The vocabulary word of COVID-19 is it's the pivot.

Exactly. It's taking my entire team and helping them pivot. It's different for almost everyone. Everybody's inside, and we used to meet people in person. Not everybody's an Instagram influencer! Some people are coffee shop people—they like to meet people in person! I can't tell you how many cups of coffee I have had building my business, but now they're *virtual coffees*. PIVOT. On my website, I actually made a page called "Virtual Coffee with Victoria". *I have my cup of coffee, and you have your cup of coffee and let's meet on Zoom*. Again, how do you figure it out? Now, the pivot is getting everybody online, and that's the wave of the future because I don't know how long this season's going to last. I do know for sure that when we come out of whatever this season is, it's going to be different.

Q: Yes, it will be different.

Now I'm focusing on trying to figure out what that is going to look like and how I can help my team be best prepared for this new reality. To get them online, help them get a website, get them comfortable with Zoom, Facebook lives—help them learn to build in a different way. It's not, *Oh my gosh, I can't build my business anymore because, you know, my kids are home.* Well, guess what? My daughter was sitting on my lap for part of this interview. People all around the world have seen my daughter sitting on my lap while I'm having meetings. That's just the new normal. She is not my excuse. She is my WHY. She is watching me. How did mommy respond to the pandemic? Was she fearful and retreated? Or was she bold and stepped up her game to serve? How do I want her to remember this season?

Q: There's a lot of people thinking, How does she do that? How does she start her business while traveling around the world? So, give me some tips. For anyone who is sitting thinking, I want to start my business, I don't know what I want to do. What would you tell them to do first?

The first thing I would say is wherever you are in the world, now is the time. This is the greatest time to start a business. It's not too late, and it's not too soon. It is just perfect, right now. *Don't hesitate.* That's number one. Number two, what fires you up? What lights you up? What gets you out of bed in the morning? What do you talk about that you really start talking faster - *with passion*? I was talking to a young man yesterday, and I was doing a kind of a health coaching call. We got onto the gut microbiome, and I was just getting all fired up, and he was like, "Wow, you really know a lot about this." Yeah... that's ONE of my things. You can be passionate about several things!

What excites you? Is it cooking? Is it gardening? Is it healthy? Is it fitness? What is the thing that makes you just get energized when you're speaking about it? Monetize your passion! Then it doesn't feel like work—it feels like FLOW.

Q: Yes, that's right.

When I am talking to people about their health or their business, I am just jazzed, and it does not feel like work to me. I know that I'm in perfect alignment with what I am doing, because I live in flow. If you are a makeup person and you love making women feel better about themselves -do that If you like helping people with their health—do that. That's the first thing. It is figuring out what fires you up. The second thing is, I am a big believer in scheduling your success. You cannot, I am sorry, but you cannot join a company or start a company then go, *Okay, where is it? Where's my success?*

I tell people, you don't need a to-do list. You need a calendar. Then obey your calendar. You schedule your success. Everything you need "to-do" should be in your calendar. Do you know I have "getting dressed" in my calendar? If I don't put it in there, it's not going to happen. I'll just start working, and then I get all fired up, and then all of a sudden the day's gone and I never got dressed. Whatever it is, you can write out your to-do list, but put it in your calendar, and then obey your calendar. That way, your to-do has a time to actually get done.

If you need to get your business license, or you need to call 20 people, or if you need to practice teaching a class, put it in your calendar. Then you'll sleep better because you know when it's going to happen. I don't lay in bed and worry about, *Oh, when am I going to make those calls? When am I going to write that content?*

When am I going to…? I don't, because I scheduled the time to do it in my calendar, and it's got a block of time when it will happen. To-do lists can sit there and collect dust. Those are dangerous things, in my book. Scheduling the time TO-DO it is the key!

Q: Victoria, this has been great. I would also go to her website, it's OYLwithoutboundaries.com.
O-Y-L is "Own Your Life." Physically, emotionally, spiritually, and financially. Take personal responsibility and *own your life*. Create your future.

Q: That is really what it's all about. Victoria specializes in helping people start a business and then also build a business. If you're interested in just learning more about what she does, I know she has a link on her OYLwithoutboundaries.com to connect with her. Reach out, connect with her, ask her questions. She's great. Victoria, thank you so much for coming on.
Such an honor to be here. My hope is that you are encouraged & empowered to step into your greatness.

CHAPTER 10:

"Building habits that support Self-care, Healthy Living, and Career Growth"

with Karissa Williams

———————————————

I AM REALLY excited to talk to my next guest. She is a health and wellness expert. She's a certified life, health and mindset coach. She's just a bona-fide badass. When I started talking to her, we just connected on the whole boss vibe. I love what she's doing. The boss babe and creator of 365 Daily Hustle.

Q: I am so excited to have you here, Karissa. How are you doing?

I'm doing fantastic, and I'm so excited to be on your "Women with a Vision" show.

Q: You've been coaching for quite a while. I used to be a health and wellness coach, but never with such intention as you. Tell me a little bit about how you started coaching.

My whole mission for the last 10 years has really been to empower, inspire, and motivate women to live their best life. I have gone through what so many of my clients are going through, and I have made it my life's work to help these women BossUp and rise above their situation. Back in the day, I looked like a very fun-loving, successful go-getter who quite honestly had her shit together. I was respected in my community and in my career, I had two awesome kids, and a husband who loved and supported me. But on the inside, it was totally different.

As someone who has experienced lots of childhood trauma, you can imagine that when I met my ex-husband at 19 years old, we had lots of things to work through. I had zero confidence, lots of self-doubt, and tons of old beliefs to let go of.

Fast forward a few years… We got married, we bought a cute little house, I started working for my mom again, we have a beautiful daughter. I thought life was pretty good. For the first time in years I was happy, I mean who wouldn't be.

But over the years I found myself taking care of everyone and everything except for me. I didn't want to focus on how bad I was still hurting on the inside, and instead I found happiness and joy in mentoring others and raising my babies. I wanted to be the best mom, wife, friend, employee, daughter, and sister that I could be. And I lost sight of being the best version of me.

Q: A lot of women are in that place or have been in that place. I'm not sure if it's a gender thing, but we tend to take care of everyone else. In your case, where do you think this comes from?

I think it comes from old childhood wounds. I watched my mom work herself to death and prove her self-worth through helping others. Almost sacrificing all family time for her business and, for her bridal shows. Anything she touched turned to liquid gold—except for our family. We were a family that was very broken. I don't have a ton of memories with my mom because she was always working in and on her business. She was bossing up, herself, which I can respect. That's exactly where I get my work ethic from. The second biggest lesson that my mom taught me, is if you work hard anything is possible. That mindset and hustle has been ingrained in me. I think that it's the story I created, that in order to be successful I have to be, *Go, go, go, go, go.* Quite honestly, if I'm not burning out and not extremely busy, then who am I? What is my worth? At the end of the day, I struggled with work-life balance, and it affected me in so many areas of my life.

In a matter of 3 years I went from weighing 120lbs to over 213lbs. I was overweight, embarrassed, and ashamed of my body and it was starting to take its toll on my life. I hated the person in the mirror, and I coped with these feelings with food, booze, cigarettes, and work.

I had a life changing moment in Germany, I was sitting in a doctor's office and I was told that for my height and weight that I was considered obese. Talk about a punch right to the gut. I knew I was overweight, and I hated the way I looked but I never considered myself to be obese.

When I got home, I lit a cigarette and huffed and puffed my entire afternoon away. I thought that if I could just go to bed, I would wake up feeling better and forget it all ever happened.

It turns out that when you have a life changing moment in a doctor's office, you wake up feeling the exact same way. But, instead of hate and embarrassment, I felt different, I felt empowered in a weird way. I got up just like any other morning. I walked my son to the bus stop, stopped by my friend Jamie's house for the daily gossip, smoked about 8 cigarettes, and drank at least 1 pot of coffee.

When I got back home.... I sat on the couch and I looked over at a picture of my mom, and for the first time in my entire life I saw just how heavy she was. I saw all 320lbs of her, I saw her battle with cancer, I saw her diabetes, I saw her quality of life or the lack thereof. And in that moment, I said to myself... Karissa, you are better than this, you need to get your life back on track, and that from that moment on I decided to raise my standards....and BossUp. I promised myself that day that I would take better care *of my body*.

Q: Right. Was she the first person who was that blunt with you?

Yes, this doctor was super blunt and honest with me.

Don't get me wrong, at first, I was upset and angry with her, but, then I realized that I needed a reality check. I ended up going back to the doctor's office and apologizing for my behavior and then I thanked her for giving me this honest truth.

Q: How long ago was this?
Let's see, I started my weight loss journey in 2010.

Q: Yeah. That aha moment created a transformation for you. So then what happened?
All I knew at the time was that I needed to eat less, eat cleaner, and move my body again. Also, I knew that I would need some help and accountability with my goals. So, I went to some neighbors and asked if they wanted to join me at the gym. I asked if they would watch Sara while I went to the gym. I also asked my mom who I called every day to help hold me accountable to my goals.

You see, I wanted to be around for my kids, I wanted to be able to have the energy to keep up with my kids, and I also wanted to look and feel good in body so that I would feel more confident around my husband and friends.

Day by day, week by week, I dragged my ass to the gym even though I hated every moment of it at first.

Not only did I start to lose the weight that year, but, I also quit smoking. I became a master of habit change. Years later, I realized that losing all of that weight still didn't make me truly happy.

Q: A lot of people struggle with making changes. You're saying that this weight is not about the weight and it's not about the food or eating. What did you discover that it was for you? What did it mean?

During my weight loss journey, I discovered so much about myself. I discovered that being healthy isn't all about a number on the scale, it isn't all about lifting weights or countless hours on the cardio machines, it's not even about eating all that chicken and sweet potatoes.

You see, being healthy is all about living life to the fullest. Living a life full of self-love, positive energy, freedom and playing BIG. It's about accepting who you are, and rocking the skin you're in, matter what others think. It's about letting go of old beliefs so that you can truly live life to the fullest.

Q: I always liken physical weight to emotional weight and to psychological weight. It shows up on the outside. It's something about protecting yourself from some pain that you haven't dealt with. It's about something way deeper than you think it is. Especially if you're at the obese stage, and you keep piling it on. You can't figure out how to let it go. You have to actually do the work.

Yeah, you do. I believe that you must hustle and work hard for your goals. You can wish and pray for your life to turn around or you can take action and BossUp. That is what I love about coaching, not only can a coach help you lose weight, but we can also help you work on your inner game. Coaching is true personal development and I love it.

By the time I got back into the states I had gone from 213lbs to 165lbs. I was feeling great and ready to lose the next 10lbs. We were in North Carolina visiting my husband's family when I got a call from my family. They told me that mom was in the hospital and that her cancer was really kicking her ass. We packed up as soon as we could, and we started the 17-hour drive back to Nebraska. We made it to St. Lewis before I realized that mom was not going to make it and as the PR of her estate, I had to make the call to let her go.

It was a tough and stressful week for all of us. When I got home, I jumped straight into planning her funeral. Losing my mom was tough, but it reminded me that I must continue to work hard and lose the weight. So, I joined a local gym, I kept eating clean, and I stuck to the habits that worked for me.

Q: Yeah. It's a never-ending battle because if you're used to dealing with stress in a certain way. Then you tend to go right back to what's comfortable for you too. What do you think in your life was your biggest hurdle to overcome?

Coaching is crazy and, what I mean by that is, when you are allowed the space to dream and get curious about your life without judgement so many crazy things can unfold for you, and holy cow, life transformations and shifts can happen.

Looking back over the last 5 years, I would have to say that it was the decision to walk away from my 14-year marriage. When I discovered that my heart was not in my marriage anymore, I decided to move on from it. It has been one of the toughest things for me to do so far. I mean, who leaves someone who has supported them mentally, emotionally, and physically. But, this girl did. During a coaching session, I realized that I wasn't truly happy... and that I was not being my true authentic self. Don't get me wrong, there were lots of times of happiness, joy, and love. But in the end my heart was not in it. And that isn't fair for anyone. Plus, it's my job as a mama to show my kids what a loving relationship looks like.

When you get a divorce, everything changes—your finances, your parenting, your relationships, self-love, even your own identity. It's been 15 years since I have been a single mama, but I have never felt more loved, supported, and happy than I do right now. If you are wondering how I made such a huge decision, I think that you have to cut through the BS and get really clear on what you want in life. Making that decision was the biggest thing that I needed to do so that I could BossUp.

When people ask me, what went wrong in my marriage I tell them that we just grew apart. Honestly, I was excelling. I'm a real go-getter, I'm a hustler, and I allowed my career and community to get the better version of me. When I came home, I was always irritable and stressed-out. I was dumping everything on my husband. My kids got a crappy version of me, and I was always yelling at them the minute I opened the door. "Why aren't the shoes in the cubby?" "Can anyone do dishes in this house besides me?" Looking back at this period in my life, I am definitely not proud of the mama that I was.

I'm often asked how I can stay positive and optimistic

when I'm facing a huge obstacle, a stressful situation, or even a devastating disappointment.

The truth is .... Yes, I do get down, and I do feel discouraged. And yes I do hit rock bottom, but after that wave of emotions pass, I remind myself that I'm going through this challenging time because there is some skill, experience, or a person that I'm meant to meet. I would not be where I am today had I not gone through such tough and painful moments.

That simple reframing, restores my faith and re-assures me that I'm exactly where I am meant to be in life.

The biggest lesson that I took away is that I can't let my hunger for building my business get the best version of me. I have learned that the relationships in my life must come first. At the end of the day, I can't snuggle up to my business. So, when you find your best friend and partner in life hold onto them because at the end of the day, that's all that really matters.

Nothing makes me happier than to have someone in my corner supporting and loving me at the end of the day. It just has to be the right partner.

Q: Yes. It's very important. You have to give to the people. The people supporting you are important to the whole thing.

Absolutely. That's one of the keys to my success—having a tribe. At the end of the day, I can't do it alone. I feel like I'm a superhero some days, but sometimes I have to hang up the cape and just be real. Some days, I need to cry it out and ask for help. That's really how I found my niche. The women I love working with are stressed-out career-focused *mamas* that have their priorities a bit mixed up. I help these women create better work-life balance leaving them feeling happy, healthy, and more accomplished.

Q: Yes, it does. You have to go through the fire in order to turn back. I would say I work with myself 10 or 20 years ago; that's who I work with because I can see who I was.

Yeah. Workaholic mama's that just have their priorities mixed up. I loved the hustle, and at times I have allowed it to consume me. And, that my friend, is not healthy.

Q: Yes. I think it makes so much sense why you call yourself 365 Daily Hustle because the woman who is attracted to that is going to be your avatar.

For sure, I love working with other fear-facing, go-getting, career mamas.

Q: That's right. How do you stay motivated? In order to give, you have got to keep filling your cup.

100%! In order to be the best version of me I've got to fill my cup first. You see self-care is another key to my success. I'm an ambassador for self-care. It's one of my core values and pillars in my coaching programs. But, I love talking about motivation. There are so many different directions that I could get into here, and I could tell you all about the awesome tools that help me stay motivated. But, in my opinion, motivation will eventually run out. There are times in our life where you can lose your way and can get stuck in a serious rut. I work with lots of women that have lost their way and are stuck in a serious rut.

How do you get out of a rut and relight the fire within? How do you get motivated again once your motivation has run out? How can you create mental toughness so that you can push past the hard times and develop an unstoppable game plan for success?

The truth is... everyone experiences struggles. I don't care if you work the drive through line, or you're the most successful person in the world, you will go through some tough and challenging times.

I stay motivated because I have built what I call "The Reset Button", this button is built on "aha" moments, past failures, and life lessons. When life gets you down, you must learn to lean in, and embrace everything that you have learned, which includes connecting with your WHY and long-term vision. It includes leaning into your tribe for support and encouragement. It means focusing on the daily wins and staying positive. But most importantly it involves taking care of yourself and listening to your heart.

Early on in my coaching career, I was struggling with finding clients. I started to doubt my ability to even be a coach. I remember thinking, did I just leave my corporate career behind for this? Am I crazy?

All these fearful thoughts started entering my mind. Honestly, I doubted every decision that I made and that stressed me out even more. I had lost my focus and drive, and my motivation was running low. With so much additional stress in my life, I found myself working more, sleeping less, feeling low energy, eating crappy, and hitting the snooze button more often. I started to recognize my behaviors and emotions, and I realized that I was in a serious "rut".

When I am feeling stressed-out and overwhelm the first thing I do is "Hit the Reset", this is a 5-step process and it goes something like this…

Step #1   Step back and Reflect, I ask myself… What is challenging me right now?

Step #2   What is one thing that I can do right now that would help me get through this?

Step #3   Who can I reach out to for help?

Step #4   What do I need to let go of in order to feel better?

Step #5   What are 5 things that I love about my life?

This is your WHY and will help you stay motivated.

Q: Yes, I can relate to every single step. We all have ups and downs. You got to step back, reset, and find what's motivating you. I remember how crappy I felt. You see, resilience is my superpower, having resilience has given me the ability to bounce back after every setback, only making me mentally, physically, and emotionally stronger.

When I look back at my life, I have a lot of childhood trauma, teenage bullshit, and major life setbacks. I have learned to view these setbacks and crappy moments in life as lesson and wins, because I would not be who I am today had I not BossedUp and found a way to push through.

My past stories don't define me, they only motivate me to empower, inspire, and educate others to live their best life. I enjoy teaching and coaching others how to BossUp and live their best life.

Q: What will you tell a woman who's at that place right now? We're in a challenging time and people are scared. I'm talking to people, and they want to get into a cocoon. They want to wrap themselves up in a blanket. What will you tell a boss woman right now? Some tips for her to boss up when it gets tough. When you're worried about everything, or you're worried about money. Where's my next client going to come from and how am I going to handle all this stuff? What would you say?

My four biggest tips to any boss or boss in the making…

Follow your heart. Every decision that I've made in the last 10 years has been made from a place of love. When you can cut out the BS of the world, the opinions, the what-ifs, and the *how am I going to get there's? And you* just make a decision from your heart. You will never be steered wrong, that I promise you.

Say yes to more self-care, healthy habits, and balance. Give yourself permission to say yes and have fun! Being a career-focused mama is like being a superhero, and even superheroes have to reset, readjust, and refocus on what's most important. Without a healthy mind, body, and spirit, who can we really take care of, honestly? How much can we even really achieve before we're burnt-out? How far can we go on the tank if it's constantly empty? So, take care of yourself always!

Be relentless when it comes to living your best life. So, play big and be courageous! Don't be afraid to let go of what holds your back.

My last tip comes from a lesson that my mom taught me. 9 years ago, I buried my mom, and with her death she taught me that life is short. You never know when you will leave this world, so you had better enjoy the life you're living today.

Q: My mom gave me the same gift before she passed as well. She gave me two gifts. One: I don't care about what anybody else thinks. So, I just do what I got to do. Two is: Life is short.

You are 100% right; life is short and other people's opinions aren't any of your concerns. Even if I lived to be 100 years old, I want to leave a certain legacy behind. I don't want to be remembered for being a successful but stressed-out mama who never made enough time for her family. I want to be remembered for being a great coach who helped lots of women. I want to be remembered for the deep love I showed my family, friends, and community. I want to be remembered as the coach who impacted so many lives.

Q: Karissa, I have just so enjoyed you. Girl, this is amazing. I know someone who's reading this is going to get inspired, empowered, and feel like they can really. Not only live the next day but have some sense of direction and purpose, and know that we all have thought we all are a boss. We all have it in us. We just have to look inside and take care of ourselves and take care of each other. I'm just so happy that you took some time out to spend with us today.

When you presented me with this opportunity, I was like.... Hell yea! *I'm fierce... I'm a bossbabe... I want to be a part of this amazing book.* But, then I realized that this book is much bigger than me. I thought that if I can share my stories with the world and I can inspire, empower and motivate just one babe to Boss Up and live her best life, then heck yes count me in.

Life is full of moments that we can either choose to stay stuck or we can choose to BossUp and live our best life.

Q: All right, Karissa, I look forward to collaborating and keeping this fun train going, girl.
Yes, ma'am, me too.

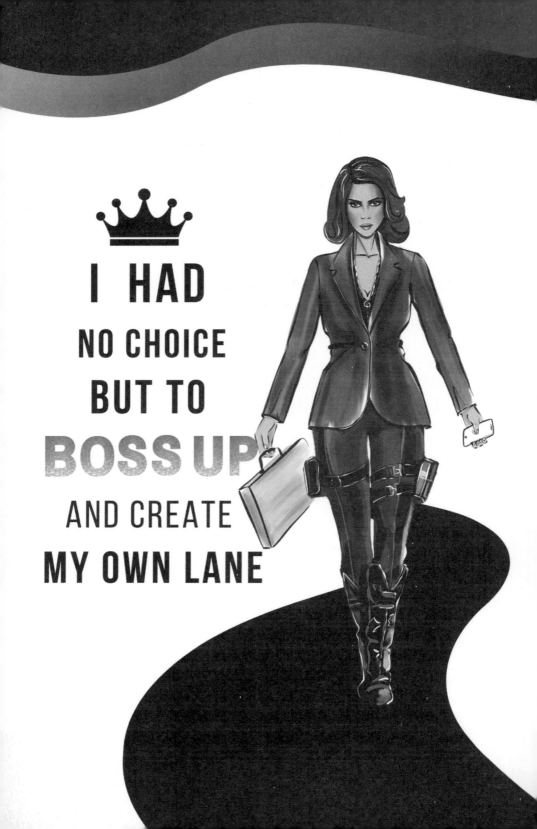

I HAD
NO CHOICE
BUT TO
BOSS UP
AND CREATE
MY OWN LANE

SECTION 4:
Women Who BossUp in Business

I am no finance expert. I can truthfully say I don't particularly enjoy math. But over years of trial and error, I have learned a lot. There are some business fundamentals that women entrepreneurs need to know. Money is not bad. Wanting money is not evil. Wanting a lot of money is not terrible. Hurting people for profit is bad. Creating a profitable business is good.

Money gives you choices and opportunities to create the life you want and give to whatever you cause you want to support. When you understand the fundamentals, you can start making the change that makes the difference.

CHAPTER 11:

"Build a successful personal brand online"

with Jasmine Kratz

═══════════════════════════════════════

THIS WOMAN FOUND me online in my group Woman with Vision International. She is from Australia and was coming through LA. We met up and have become fast friends since then and do a lot of collaborating together. I'm really excited to introduce her.

Q: Jasmine, how are you?

I'm awesome. Thank you so much for having me. I'm having an amazing day.

Q: Jasmine, you are a boss. I know this for sure because we work on a lot together. You have a business called Inspired Impact that you established back in 2015, with a mission to become the best marketing agency for entrepreneurs, to build their brand online without technical overwhelm. Tell me a little bit about how you came up with this idea and what got you started.

Sure, I'd love to share. So back in 2014, I had been working in the corporate world for nearly 20 years. I was working really long hours managing hotels and resorts with my husband. My daughter was very little and I was just going through the process of, you know, there's got to be more for me. I was 30 and I felt like 50, and I really wanted to be able to have my own business and work my own hours and do things for myself. So back then, I sort of fell into the network marketing industry and I started to learn that there was a way to make an income online.

There was something I could do from home around the family and, at that time, around my corporate role as well. And so, I dived into that whole realm of entrepreneurship and how to make an income online. And like most people in that space, I felt very overwhelmed with all of the choices and all of the things I needed to piece together and how it all works. And so, as someone with a marketing degree and a major in information systems and business, I was like, if I'm struggling with all this then how are people who have no idea going to be able to piece all of this together?

You know, I have a product and I have a business model that I can do that's not just face-to-face and that I can do online to leverage my time, but how can I stand out from the crowd? How can I differentiate myself? Five years ago, personal branding wasn't really a key term that anyone really talked about. But the fact is leading with value and sharing things—that, as part of your transformational story, allow you to stand out from everyone else who might be selling the same product or service—is obviously key to attracting more people, more customers, more clients.

And so I really went down that path of learning those skills for myself and being able to then apply that to the business I had at the time. Obviously, my business has evolved and grown over those years and now offers different services and opportunities. However, the principles are still the same: build a personal brand and then you can share whatever it is that is on your heart at the time and whatever your skill set is that you can monetize. So that's really where Inspired Impact was born. It was that opportunity to brand who I am and what I have and my skill set, and then I just started attracting other people. They saw what I did back in the day in network marketing. It was the system to do things a certain way and I wanted to be unique and do it my way. Just break the mold. And I thought, *Well, this is how I'm going to roll, just to see how it works.*

Q: I didn't realize until now that we both have that background. So, do you think network marketing is a good place to start?

Yes, a hundred percent. A lot of the clients I serve and support now are leaders in the network marketing industry. And helping them to be able to brand themselves and stand out from the crowd and attract their ideal team and customers is how it evolved for me. Because I had a team at the time and they all wanted to know how I was doing, what I was doing, and that turned into Inspired Impact. Being able to offer the services that I now do to help more people shine online and have their own online brands and services.

Q: That's really cool, but where did that start? We both have a degree in marketing. What inspired you to go into that?

I think, if you take it right back to when I was younger, my parents had their own businesses. And I, from a very early age, was just really, really good at troubleshooting, really good at finding solutions to problems and thinking outside of the box to figure out how we could do things differently. I started working pretty young in the family business. I've always been very creative. I was never going to be a graphic designer, but I love visuals and I love design. Personal Branding flows from my love shopping and clothes and all those sorts of fashion. But I think, for me, choosing a business management degree, majoring in marketing information systems communication, at university, gave me the understanding of systems and automation. I did my four years of my degree and I was working full time already in the corporate world.

Then being able to apply the things I was learning at university in a real-life business really helped me, especially all those assignments. Everyone else was having to come up with fictitious businesses and ideas to create their assignments. And I was doing it in real life. So the things I was learning, I was actually able to apply and support and help those hospitality and tourism businesses that I was working in. I think that was where that passion came from, because I could actually see the things I was learning and implementing having a positive effect in someone's business. From the age of 18 or 19, I was a manager running other people's hotels and resorts and having an impact. I was pouring my heart and soul into this business, but it wasn't my own.

And so, from that drive and dedication came the thinking, *You know, I can take things only so far because it's not my business, not my money.* I could only do so much as a manager, so I wasn't really able to step into really making the impact I wanted to in my life. At the time, I didn't know that's what I was creating, but there was always this drive to have my own business, my own team, my own hours. I mean, I've probably worked more hours now than I ever would have thought. It's my passion. It's what I love to do. And so it doesn't feel like work. I think that really it stems from a young age. Seeing my family and then working in the managerial space at a young age made me realize that the success I was creating for them was what I wanted to be able to create for myself one day.

Q: Very cool. And I know it's not always easy. What are some of the obstacles you have gone through over the years of your business?

For sure, I mean, a hundred percent, it's not all the pretty pictures you've seen portrayed on Instagram and Facebook. There're a lot of hours and a lot of sacrifices that we make with our family. But for me, working from home with two kids and my husband who's also an entrepreneur with his own business, the struggles are much more worth it than ever going back into the corporate world. We've picked up and moved and traveled across the state. Some people don't even believe it, but I, at one point, actually traveled around Australia in my caravan for two years, working and running my network marketing business. Some people said, "You are absolutely nuts! You traveled in the caravan with a one-year-old?" But it was the best time of our lives. Seriously, that was freedom to me. It wasn't about having the big flashy house and all of those nice things—which, of course, we love having—but having that freedom to be with my family and be with my daughter when she was so young was the best thing we could have done. And she still remembers that time, and so I didn't feel it was crazy, but it was definitely interesting. That was definitely a hurdle we overcame.

Q: Well, I think that's great.

Yeah, and then we settled, and then we travelled it again when I was pregnant with my youngest for about three months. And because my business was online, it wasn't affected. No one really even knew that's what I was doing. Once I had my phone and Wi-Fi and laptop, I was free. That was the freedom I was always looking for, to be able to travel and do what I wanted to do. I mean, it certainly hasn't come without sacrifices, you know Mummy does spend a lot of time sitting at her computer, but I also get to go to all the school things. I also get to travel for months to give my kids the opportunities that I could never have done if I was still working a 9-5. So I feel very grateful for the life that I have created through my business, but it certainly hasn't come without the struggles some months not knowing where the next client is going to come from, Or how am I going to pay for my team? You know, all of those are things that you go through as a business owner, but somehow we just boss up and keep on going. We just make it happen.

Keep on showing up and the universe aligns. Lead with value, lead with service, be of service, and be here to support. And they just show up.

Q: They show up, yes. What would you say your biggest hurdle has been for you to overcome?

I think, in the early days, it was definitely shiny object syndrome. It was, who do I follow? Whose advice do I take? What's the next step? How do I piece all of this together because there are so many working parts to having an online business? I mean, we could talk about that all day, but like, how do I price my offers? What offers does the market want? What platforms should I build my website on? What about social media? It's endless, the things you could be doing. And how do you know what the right path is, from potentially being stuck in the corporate world, to actually replacing your income and then thriving and doubling and tripling it, and then being featured in magazines and books and having clients everywhere all over the world? What are those little micro steps you should be taking?

And so, for me, I definitely went down that rabbit hole of spending a lot of time and money in a place of, *Am I doing the right thing? What's the next step for me?* But I think it comes down to trusting your gut, finding someone who has the results you want, learning from them and bridging that gap. Shorten that space for you so that you don't have to make all the mistakes they made. Learn the fastest route to success, and that's where having a coach and investing in yourself come in. You have to invest in your business and invest in yourself before you see the results, and you just have to trust the process. So I went through all of that, spent a lot of time and a lot of money on every course and every downloadable and all the things that taught me. That's been my path to success, anyway. And everyone's path is different, but I think that was the biggest thing, Try to stay laser focused, find someone who has those results you want, follow their advice, implement it, and just keep on going and going. Put one foot in front of the other and trust yourself, trust your gut.

We each have a unique entrepreneurial journey and some people, friends, and family won't understand what you're doing. They don't have the entrepreneurial mindset that we have. I've been very, very lucky and grateful that I have an extremely supportive husband and family that have always believed in me and have always said, "You know, baby, you've got this, I trust you and you know what you're doing. Just do your thing." Even if they don't understand what my thing is, they have supported me, and for that I am eternally grateful. And I think that if you don't have that around, you find it. Find the community or find those online BFFs who are going to be there as your cheerleaders because you need them.

Q: You need them because they get it. That really is everything.

Yeah, it is. A hundred percent. Because otherwise, it can be very lonely. It can be a lonely journey a lot of the time, however I do love the peace and quiet, but I do work on my own most of the time. It's not a busy office where you have a coffee machine and you chat and all those things. Most of us are boss moms juggling homeschooling and a whole lot of things and we connect and have the conversations that keep you going on messenger or whatsapp but its the connection with like minded souls that keeps you grounded.

Q: Oh yes, and that brings me to a whole new topic. Right now, it's craziness with Covid-19 and lockdowns, being the homeschool teacher as well as everything else. How is that?

I have a five-year-old and I have a 13-year-old, so we're dealing with grade one and grade eight schoolwork. As I said, my husband has his own business as well. So yeah, this time's been very interesting. It's been challenging. I think props to everyone who's getting through this in isolation together and running their businesses because we could just throw our hands up and go, okay, business is on hold for three months, I can't deal. But no, we're just stepping up even more, bossing up, helping even more people, pulling all-nighters to get everything done. I mean, it's an interesting time, but I think it's where leaders are really going to shine, where diamonds are made. Because it would be very easy to just say I'm going to pause, I'm just going to watch Netflix and chill, and my business will still be there in three months.

But no, this whole new wave of people who now need our help, the clients we have served who already have online businesses, they're having to pivot, they're having to change. And so, for me, I've been busier than ever in supporting my community and my existing clients. They might've already had an online presence, but their actual core businesses are still face-to-face, or brick-and-mortar stores and services, whether it was massage or health or something else, but they've had to pivot. We're putting in a lot of work to take what they were doing face-to-face and bringing that online. And now there are new referrals of people who are saying, "Okay, well, I've lost my job," or, "I can't work from the office anymore. I need the fastest way to get online and start making money to support my family."

And so, I'm stepping into a whole other realm I didn't think I was ready for, but it just threw me in. "Okay, I'm ready to lead you and show you the way." It doesn't have to be overwhelming. There is so much uncertainty right now, and people are already in a state of overwhelm with what's going on at home, let alone figuring out how to start a business online. And so, that's what I'm really passionate about and why I'm working crazy hours and doing the things I've been doing. I'm so passionate about helping anyone who needs my help to do that, to bring their brand online, and not have the tech piece be the stumbling block because that's what I see every day. "What platform do I use? How do I connect this to that? Do I need this? Do I need that?" And so that's what I live and breathe now, and it's a very simple process for me, but it's not for most when they start to dive into that.

Q: "What do I do?" I know, I see it every day too. Well, I love this. I love what you're doing and that you are also a part of our book, Women Who BossUp. I'm so excited about it.

Q: And you also were in an online magazine called YMag featuring eight female change-makers for 2020. Tell me a little bit about that.
Yeah, so that was really exciting. It was released last month April 2020. YMAG is for a community of women who are purpose-driven to be the best versions of themselves.

YMag® is an authentic, real, inclusive brand that empowers women unlike any other magazine. And is specifically for female entrepreneurs. It's a place to be inspired. It's a place for you to read other women's journeys and what they've been through to get to where they are today. So to be featured as one of the eight change-makers for 2020 was a real honor and something that I was really, really proud of. Yeah, just being able to share my story with others and give them that inspiration that they can do it too. I was a mum of two who was stuck in the corporate world as an assistant and not living my purpose . I really changed my life and built this business from scratch, and now I meet people all over the world and get to travel and run my events and retreats. It's pretty special to be able to share that story.

Q: Awesome. If you want to keep up with Jasmine, definitely go to her website inspiredimpact.com.au and check her out. She's amazing. I look forward to doing many, many more things with you in the future.

Me too, thank you so much, Tam. I really appreciate it and value the connection and, yeah, so awesome that we got to meet in person as well.

"Today is not your

forever reality"

—CLARA CAPANO

CHAPTER 12:

"BossUp as a Sleep Specialist"
with Summer Hartman

═══════════════════════════════════

I AM REALLY excited today to be talking with my next guest who is incredible. Her name is Summer Hartman. I became aware of what she does because she's one of the Boss Ladies who was a part of our community, Women with Vision, and I am amazed by what she has created.

Q: Summer, how are you doing?
I'm good. I'm staying as healthy as possible right now and staying indoors.

Q: Yes, it's such an interesting time. Where are you calling me from?

I live outside of Phoenix, Arizona, just about 20 minutes, in a small town called Maricopa. I don't want to live in the city, so we chose a small town.

Q: I'm excited to talk to you. First of all, you have been ranked one of the top 200 best sleep consultants by www.tuck.com. You have a company called Summer's Sleep Secrets. What got you started doing that?

My original brand was Sleeping Sweet Peas, and I got started as a newborn care specialist back in 2007. I interviewed for an agency and they said if I had been a nanny for more than three years, they would hire me to work nights with newborns. So I fit the bill. I have been a nanny since I was 18 years old. It just took off and I have not stopped. And I've had some wild, wild cases.

Q: I have become more aware of this because my girlfriend just had a baby. She hired a live-in nanny and sleep consultant.

Just to clarify, a night nurse means they have to be an RN. So they're actually considered night nannies, newborn care specialists, or infant care specialists. Just as an FYI. People always get irritated.

So I started as a nanny in 1996. I was recruited by a lawyer who worked in the White House under Bill Clinton's administration. I worked with high-level clients from outside of the country as well as this lawyer's children as a live-in. It was high pressure with high demand.

Q: Wow. Tell me about being a sleep correspondent for NPR news and parent.com?

Yes. Those came about through Twitter, because I got really popular on Twitter during a six-month job. The parents didn't want any sleep training, so I had to hold the baby all night long and I had to stay awake. I built my Twitter account during that six months. I got a lot of experience and a lot of people reaching out through Twitter. That's how that happened.

Q: You have been doing this basically your whole life. Can you tell me a little bit about that?

My parents moved us around a lot when we were young. My dad was a pro bowler, so he would do tournaments in Vegas, Seattle, wherever the big tournaments were. So whenever there was a baby in the bowling alley, I gravitated to them. I was holding babies from like eight years on. My parents had my brother when I was eight years old. Then my parents bought a bowling alley in Idaho when I was 12 and I became the city babysitter. Everyone came bowling, they picked me up from the bowling alley from like 12 to 14. As soon as I turned 15, I was driving to the houses to babysit. I've never not had babies. This is my longest period right now where I've basically been quarantined for the last three months. I haven't had a baby.

Q: Maybe, since you are quarantined, you will end up having another baby. Or your business might go boom, right after this quarantine is over.

Haha…maybe.

Q: Because you have so much experience and, obviously, you love babies, what inspired you to start your business the way it is now?

It evolved over time. My main focus for 10 years was working nights and taking care of babies overnight as well as supporting families. I would work seven nights a week. I didn't have a lot of time to do anything else. Then, around 2014, I got sick and I realized I was losing my memory. So I started to write down all my memories. I also felt like there was a lack of training in our industry on how to properly do sleep training. There's a method. There is a reason behind what we do as NCS that gets babies to sleep through the night by 12 weeks. And it wasn't taught in any of the classes at that point. So I took all the knowledge I had and wrote a book during that time. It took me six months to write it.

Q: Did you feel you would lose it if you didn't write it down?

My brain wasn't functioning at full capacity as I wasn't getting the proper amount of oxygen, so I decided I had to write it down just in case I passed away. I felt like my family had history, my daughter could work, and they could also sell the book.

Q: Tell me a little bit about your illness.

We don't really know. It was triggered by a medication I took for weight loss. It was a trial drug and it was also partially for diabetics only. They didn't tell me that at the time. I wasn't diabetic at the time.

It triggered an autoimmune distress in me. Instead

of going to my brain, it closed off my airway. Over the next five years, my trachea started closing very gradually till it came to a point that when I walked, I'd have to stop breathing. Or I would have to hold my breath in order to talk. For a really long time, I had to fake it with clients. I told them I had asthma.

I went to the hospital over 20 times, over the next several years. They did a normal scan and said I had asthma, which wasn't true. But when I finally collapsed and went to the ER, the doctor said, "You're going to be dead by Monday, but we don't know why. We're going to put you in ICU." And I was just sitting there cross-legged like, *What the heck is going on?* I knew I was dying. I just didn't know from what. So they scoped me and they couldn't get it past the trachea. I was transferred to a different hospital and had emergency surgery to open up my airway, and it was the first time in five years that I could breathe. It was amazing. It was like being resurrected.

Q: How long ago was this?
That happened on October 31st, 2017. I've had two surgeries and I still have to have steroid injections in my throat to keep it open. So, it has not gone away. But it's just managed.

Q: Has your memory improved? Have they found a cure?
We know that there's no cure for this autoimmune response and my body will just keep attacking itself, but we know I can get surgery or a steroid injection. So I don't ever panic now. I was having panic attacks like

10 times a day because I couldn't breathe. It was scary. This virus that's going around where you can't breathe, I'm absolutely terrified because I've lived it.

Q: So how did you keep growing your company while you were sick?

I don't stop. Even when I was sick, I created my company. I still did recordings. I'd pause, try to be as smooth as possible. I did that for six weeks. I ended up throwing that out because the breathing was so bad. So I had to re-record once I could breathe again for another six weeks. Then I gathered more information and had to do it again. I've spent so much time building on my company, but that's what it takes. I never stopped building my company. I just kept doing it. That's what kept me going. I could have easily laid in bed and just died.

Q: This is why you are a Boss. There really is so much to be learned by what you're saying. Of course, you have to take care of yourself.

It's not overnight. I hate people who think any of this is easy and it's going to happen overnight. Even if it did, you're not going to succeed because you didn't put all the backing into it. I'm happy to keep working to grow it, because I don't need to make a billion dollars. I just need to provide for my family. As long as you have a good mindset. This year, at tax time, my husband was really surprised that we had accumulated this much income. I didn't know either because, when you're working, you keep on chugging and money keeps on flowing.

Q: You're doing what you love, you're passionate about what you're doing and that's all that really matters. Another thing I find interesting is how you've overcome several obstacles. Tell me about the major car accident.

Yes. So, I was going to see a client who had put their baby in hospice, and I had been with her since she was born. So I was just mentally not there that day. I said goodbye to her, and I went to the grocery store. As I was walking across the parking lot, probably about 10 feet from the front door of the grocery store, a car decided to go around another car and he didn't look forward.

He threw me about five feet from his vehicle and hit me directly at about eight miles an hour. I did like a whole 180 in the air. I landed on my left side and he shattered my bone down the middle. It was a bad break. I've now got this obstacle right from December 29th. I was in the hospital for six days and I had surgery and my airway was impacted. My lungs won't inflate. It was very, very scary.

Q: Through all of that, you were still working on your website and working on your business.

Yes. I rebuilt the entire website. That's email responses, marketing responses, etc. It was so much work to build this website, but I had three months to do it. I was like, *Why not? Don't be lazy for six weeks.* The first six weeks before that, I lay and watched TV. I watched the whole series of New Girl, which I had never done because I never watched TV. It was like seven years of the series, then I started working again. I'm good. Now I can go back.

Q: You are the epitome of a woman who never gives up.
Well, you really can't. I mean, we have obstacles every day and we can be lazy. Just like the virus now. We can look at this as an opportunity or we can look at it as, "oh no, I lost my job". Well then, recreate yourself. Because you have a skill. You have something that somebody else doesn't have. Start offering that service. I cannot tell you how many times I'm telling people this. I feel like I'm talking to a wall. Whatever you're good at, start honing in. Start writing it and make it virtual. This is the time to go virtual if you're going to.

Q: Yes. It's only a problem if you make it a problem. Now you can reach people in a different way. Just take a couple deep breaths and focus on what you do. Then boss up.
And stand six feet from everybody else, haha. I think that's what sells my business the most, my courageousness through all of my troubles. A lot of people know where I came from. How sick I've been. Back in 2012, on my 35th birthday, I had a pulmonary embolism and my left lung had nine blood clots. So I have lived through quite a bit of obstacles. Every six years, I get thrown something different. But again, you pick yourself up and reinvent yourself. Now we have this break. So I have to do things virtually. I just figure out how I am going to work, but my brain doesn't stop.

Q: You are supporting a lot of parents, nannies, doulas, and sleep experts. Do you train virtually now?
I do. It's gotten to the point where I don't need to ever go into somebody's home unless they really need

it. If they just take their phone to the nursery, I can see what's in the nursery that needs to be fixed. My husband tells me I look like the Good Doctor when he's looking at a gram. That's what I do with babies. I look at the image and know instantly what needs to be done. That's where I'm at now.

Q: I love it. So, if someone is a new parent, what would you tell them to do first?
It depends on the age of the baby. You have to ask the question as a new mom, just come home from the hospital. First, we're going to just work on nursing, if that's their goal. That's the first thing I do. I tell them to first stay in and nurse for at least the first two weeks. Let's adjust your body with the baby. And then, we start working on the baby.

Q: Can you teach them that virtually?
Oh, yes. There's no reason for me to even be there. The only reason I would need to be there at that time is if I needed to actually show her how to physically lift her breast. But I can have a husband, mate, partner, or friend hold the phone up and let me see her breast through the phone. And if there's an issue, I can say it right there. It's more for the mom's comfort that they want us there.

Q: Yes. Especially when they're brand new, they're a little nervous. When you are looking for people to work with, is it the parents or the sleep care professionals?
It's both. My whole goal in rebuilding my website was to have good marketing for families because I really want to reach them. I've reached the doulas, the

newborn care specialists, and the nannies. They know my name. They know who I am and they can find me. So I really want to get into marketing with parents more. When you're a newborn care specialist, you work with a family between six weeks and three months. You're there for 12 weeks and then you move on to the next family. In a year's time, you can have four to six families, depending on the length of the contract. So it's still not that many people you're supporting. But consulting would be really ideal. I can consult a lot of families.

Q: Are you writing a parenting book?
I am. It's just going to be a booklet about the methods I use, taking what I've already written and putting it in parenting style.

Q: Well, I tell you what, Summer, you are simply a joy to talk to and very inspiring. How do we find you?
Well, thank you so much. www.summerssleepsecrets.com

"Don't live in the past thinking about the mistakes you made. Learn from them and move on. Make them as your fuel to keep going."

—TAM LUC

CHAPTER 13:

"Creating life balance with private money lending strategies"
with Jodi Vetterl

═══════════════════════════════

I AM EXCITED to share my next guest. Her name is Jodi Vetterl, all the way from Vancouver, Canada.

Q: How are you doing, Jodi?
I am great. Thanks so much for having me on your show, Tam. I absolutely love what you are doing. You are brilliant!!!

Q: Thank you so much. I love what you are doing too. Jodi is the author of a book called Beyond the Bank Success Strategies and Real Estate as a Private Lender. She also has another program called Beyond the Book, which supports authors on how they can find premium partners to collaborate with while writing their book.

Yes, it is all very exciting. The essence of both programs is taking control of our finances to create space for ourselves, so we can afford & focus on our goals, whatever they may be.

Q: I love it. Jodi is in real estate investing, which is similar to what I did in my previous life. You were also 20 years in high-tech software sales—that is where you started, right?

Yes, I worked with some of the giants, like Autodesk and ANSYS. In my last job, I was providing engineering simulation software across all physics to various engineering disciplines.

Q: Not only that, but you also have won multiple sales achievement awards, closed seven-digit deals. Several Presidents' Club trips around the world. You were really doing it and were very successful in sales in your career.

Yes. I love my job, and the reason was that the technology was so fascinating. To be working with the innovators & early adopter companies was a real privilege. Having the opportunity to go behind the curtains and witness the technology developed in my territory was made for a fascinating job.

Q: Very cool. You stayed in corporate America for a long time. Was it 20 years or 17 years that you were in corporate?

It was pretty much 20 years on the nose!

Q: Oh, wow. Were you simultaneously building your real estate portfolio at the same time?

Absolutely. When I first started working for software manufacturers, I was just touching six figures, and it blew me away that that was even available to me. I thought to myself. I am not going to mess around with this opportunity because you never know how long it will last.

I was also very interested in real estate and learning some strategies that I could effectively participate in while a sales road warrior with a vast territory.

My grandfather was quite a real estate entrepreneur. He owned commercial real estate in the town that I grew up in. It was in my blood, and I had to start somewhere, which was with a real estate investing education course. My Grandfather had long passed away before I was at the age of even looking into it. I started learning through a real estate program out of Ontario and jumped in with buying long-term, tenanted, buy and holds.

I also had the dream of fixing and flipping houses because I love designing, and my degree was in architecture. However, the reality was that I did not have the time nor space to do this being a road warrior with the whole country of Canada as my territory. I was doing over 120,000 miles in the sky a year and enjoying all of the perks from business travels and having a lot of fun, of course. Fix, and flips take time, skill, practice, systems, and, most of all, presence. Buy-and-hold, long-term real estate investing, with some additional strategies layered in, such as joint ventures, and rent to own models have all paid off. It has been rewarding and helped establish a solid financial foundation. If I were to do it all again, I would have played bigger in real estate over investing in mutual funds and other investments I didn't fully understand. That is hindsight, and I know looking back is pointless. I can only appreciate where I am in the present.

Q: I did that in the early 2000s—2006, 2007. Then, all of a sudden, pop. A lot of people had issues during that time. Did you experience that downturn in the economy?

Yes and no. I benefited from the crash in real estate; however, the money I had in the stock market that was managed by a financial advisor caused a tremendous amount of stress, as I was hit pretty hard with the downturn of 2008. It was tough because the decisions were to wait and hope that it bounces back or sell and cut my losses. I felt shackled, like damned if I do and damned if I don't. It was a challenging time that gave me many lessons and established my money rules, one of them being that no matter where invested, I must be able to sleep at night.

In terms of real estate, I only had Canadian properties at that time, and Canada wasn't affected the same way the US market was because the Canadian banks are stricter and, therefore, more stable. They never got involved in the "liar" loans that created the crisis. I had also bought the properties early on under a cash flowing model, and I had good tenants, so everything was fine. The opportunity came when the Canadian dollar was at par with the US dollar, and US housing was on sale.

I met this fantastic investor out of Vancouver, who had developed an incredible system buying properties West of Phoenix. She was actively flipping residential real estate with a partner realtor from Phoenix, who had also started her property management company. So she would raise capital from Canadians to buy a block of 10-12 houses from the bank sales; paint and carpet; add new appliances; and place the tenants, creating a turn-key model for Canadians to invest. I bought three houses during that time, and she mentored me through the process of setting up to own real estate in the US as a Canadian. I was lucky to have met her and been mentored by her. She now runs a multi-billion dollar company where her company, Western Wealth Capital, is the 2nd largest owner of multi-family buildings in Phoenix and has grown into other markets such as Houston, Dallas, San Antonio, and Atlanta. I continue to invest with her in those markets through her multi-family syndication.

Q: That's great learning, which has fueled what you're doing today. You finally did leave corporate America and established financial independence at the age of 46. You fulfilled a lot of different things. I want to go back even further because there's obviously a love of either investing or real estate. I know you mentioned something about your Grandfather, but tell me a little bit about what really was driving you toward real estate and investment.

There's a couple of things from when I was a kid. I grew up as a pretty independent kid. I was very pushed to persevere by my Dad. At the time, I thought, *why are you pushing me so hard?* He was the kind of guy who said, *if you're riding your bike up a hill, you don't get off your bike and walk. You push through it until you are at the top, or if you're going to run a race, you're going to pace yourself, and then sprint at the end, and give 110%.* He was the 110% guy. He put me on the boys' hockey team at age seven. I played with the boys and worked hard at it. It sparked the competitive side of me, especially competing with the boys. I always had to work harder than the boys because I was a girl; this even rang true for me throughout my high-tech career. I was still trying to get that approval from my Dad, *"Hey dad, look how hard I'm working."* It was my Dad in many ways who taught me perseverance, and my Mom taught me responsibility because she was the person managing it all—Household, job, animals, kids, sports, etc. My parents have also always been entrepreneurs and even had a laundry-mat as a side-hustle and joint-ventured with a few others in a commercial building where my Grandfather established the strategy.

Nowadays, we talk a lot about kidpreneurs, and I've got a little story. I'll share a little later about my five-year-old business partner.

So when I was a kid, my brother and I had a paper route, and my grandpa also hired my brother and me to sweep his commercial property's parking lot. We were only seven, eight, nine years old doing these jobs. I liked the paper route but didn't enjoy sweeping the parking lot at night after a long day of school and homework. It was great to make money and learn a little bit about responsibility. We also lived across the street from a golf course. My brother and older cousin would go out to collect golf balls, and I'd think, *"Hey, I want to be part of this,"* but they wouldn't let me. So I said, well, screw you, then I'm going to go to it myself. So I went in the creeks by myself and scooped up the golf balls, and then made them all shiny and pretty, put them in an egg carton, and sold them back to the golfers. I was coming home—at like 11, 12 years old—with 40, 60 bucks in my pocket, and everyone's saying, *what's going on with you?* I got a taste of entrepreneurship and building a business—and I liked it. I worked in restaurants from 15 years old to 28 years old. After high school, I worked at a bank as a bank teller and a fitness facility making fitness club sales and always had those restaurant and bar jobs. My theory strategy was to save my paychecks and live off the tips. It served well and helped me save for University and travel, which were the two things I valued most throughout my 20's. I traveled to 35 countries before I was 30 yrs old and graduated with a Bachelor of Environmental Design, Faculty of Architecture.

Q: Amazing! My Dad was also an entrepreneur, and he told us that if you know how to sell, you can always survive. He said salespeople would change the world. No—he said, a salesperson will save the world.
Selling is a fantastic skillset. You will always find work and be able to transfer this skillset. The key is to represent the products and services that you believe in while being resourceful. I learned very early on in my career that if you are good at sales and meet your targets, you will always have opportunities. Without sales, there is no money coming in to afford everything else.

Q: In terms of having an entrepreneurial spirit, tell me a little bit about your business. What do you do? I know you have your book, but what kind of business do you run?

I have created an eight week guided transformational process to financial independence by utilizing private money lending with real estate investing.

A little bit of the backstory to how this came about: my move from corporate to financial independence happened when I returned to work after my Canadian mat leave of a year and ended up with a new boss who was a former peer where our values didn't align.

I came to a realization that required a life-altering decision.

The underlying drive came down to my "Why." The stress and anxiety I was carrying from this person were affecting the way I was showing up as a Mom and a partner to my husband. It was such a journey to become a Mom, and I wasn't the Mom I wanted to be or had envisioned. I was missing those precious moments with my son being silly and fun because of the stress. I would race him to daycare and run back to my desk for the early morning conference calls. If he was sick with the daycare virus and my husband was traveling, I had to try working around that, and it was complicated to have client calls. It has become more accepting now with COVID-19 to work from home and have a child in the background of a zoom meeting, but at the time, my boss actually used that against me, stating that my family life was affecting my job, which simply wasn't right. In fact, it was my job that affected my family life because I was scrambling and stressed to make it the priority and worked hard at trying to gain his approval, which was never going to come. I will never sacrifice my well-being or my family's well-being for the approval of someone or my job. I gave away my power, and it wasn't until I realized this that I took that power back. It's a bit of a tangent I know but an essential part of my journey and lessons that brought me to the transition.

The tension between my boss and I, forced, yet inspired me to roll up my sleeves and have an honest financial reality check myself. It's something that I hadn't done for a long time. Through the exercise, I realized I had underperforming assets and locked up equity. I had already been dabbling in private money lending and saw my net worth finally growing for the first time. I was able to recognize that with some restructuring, I could access capital that would meet my goal of financial independence. And what financial freedom meant for me was the ability to leave my job where I could calm down, create space, and launch into entrepreneurship.

Once I left, I had space to write my book, Beyond the Banks, Success Strategies in Real Estate as a Private Lender. Then came the coaching program, which evolved into a scalable online course that helps action-oriented people who want to change the way they invest where they are more in control of where their money is.

My audience and students learn to understand what they are investing in. They learn to ask the right questions and understand the exits. The numbers make sense, and they can easily plan for taxes and their future.

It's a simple, accelerated, and profitable way of investing. I love it and have never looked back and seen that the systems and strategies work for others makes me super proud to be a position of knowledge and experience where I can share and make a difference for others.

It's been an enormous process. Sometimes it feels overwhelming with so many learning curves and every corner you turn. There are decisions to make that cost money, and I always have to be telling myself that it does not cost money, but rather that I'm investing in myself and my business.

Through the process of writing my book, I was introduced by my publisher, to the idea of funding the book with sponsors. I was very successful at raising well over 6-figures for my book and coaching program with premium partners where we were able to create a win-win.

The partnership program I developed evolved, and I discovered all these other areas to support the joint-partnerships, which has been truly exciting. Without incorporating the raise of capital for my business, it would have been very challenging to succeed. As authors, course creators, business-owners, we learn very quickly that it's a very costly journey. People on this journey often ask me to raise money for their book, which I don't have the bandwidth. It inspired me to create a workshop called Beyond the Book offered in small weekly group meetings over eight weeks with some one-on-one time. This way, I can help more people develop partnerships and raise money to pursue their dreams and goals. While also being able to support them one on one and dive into what they are writing about and who are their audiences. It's gratifying as I have a big passion for this.

The common thread of my business is all to do with financial independence. Helping people figure out where money can come from to support whatever they are trying to achieve.

In addition to Beyond the Banks Academy, and Beyond the Book Workshops, I am launching a podcast in 2020. The podcast will focus on multiple streams of income and different investing strategies. It's exciting because I love helping people, and what is so fun is working with people and witnessing the popcorn go off in their head when they start to shift their mindset and learn different strategies. Being part of people achieving their goals is so gratifying on a level that I had never dreamed of being a part of. Anytime doubt about what I'm doing starts to seep in for me, the universe seems to deliver a message from someone I have impacted, and it warms my heart. I'm very grateful.

Q: That's good. You took some time to start doing the work early. Now, what would you say to people that want to start now?

Start with investing in yourself. Don't be afraid to invest in education. Knowledge is power, and the more you learn and understand and put into practice, the more you will grow. Start wherever you are at and don't spend energy comparing yourself to others.

Do a financial reality check and see where your money is and how it is performing.

Make sure you understand the investments you are in and how fees and commissions are structured. There is a whole world of investing beyond the banks and countless strategies to earn money. Understand your exit strategy; in other words, what needs to happen with the investment to get your money back with interest as per the contract? Get yourself organized, figure out your monthly cost of living, and, most important, set up your goals, and have some fun with it. Be realistic with where you are at now, and what your cost of living is, and then go crazy on your goals, set the bar high! What do you want to be doing in the future? If money wasn't an issue, what would you be doing now? What are your passions? How can you help others, and how can you monetize by building a business around your passion?

Q: Yes, that's really good. What keeps you inspired to keep going no matter what? What's their biggest inspiration?

I would say there are two main inspirations. One is the people with who I surround myself. When COVID first came out, I had a couple of conversations with some realtor friends, and it just seemed like they were paralyzed by it all. Then, it scared me a little bit because I thought *this is very doom and gloom, should I be worried?* I'm in some mastermind groups, and I'm on a lot of different group calls with people who are out there with their boots on the ground and doing big things. I also work with these fantastic active investors—and it's night and day. Working with people who are so solutions-driven, where their mindset is, *challenge accepted*, let's get this done. What do we need to do? There is no problem; there are just solutions. They are hustling. I'm so impressed with them. They inspire me, they light me up, and I talk to these people daily. I have to-it's important.

Q: It's important. Life is just a puzzle, right? It's just a puzzle to be solved. You take whatever piece you have. One piece, five pieces, a hundred pieces—no matter how many pieces you have—it's just a puzzle. You work with what you have, and you go out actively looking for the other pieces.

It's about perspective. I went on a bike ride with my son—he just turned five. He's an April Fool's baby and quite the bike rider. He's been on a bike since he was under two years old. He's building up his leg strength, and he's still working on his hills and stand-ups. But sometimes he gets frustrated, and then he says, *I can't, I can't do this*. I just said to him, *no, no, no, Hunter. You don't use that word in front of Mommy. That is not a word you use in front of Mommy. It's, I can, I am, and I am Hunter B, and I can do anything*. That is his mantra when he is with me. I get him into that groove of his mantra, then, next thing you know, he's riding his bike up the hill, saying, *I can, I am. I am Hunter B. I can do anything*.

Every day I let him know that I believe in him and that I'm proud of him. He is my '*why*,' He drives me to get up and do all of this stuff. As a result, every day, he tells me he believes in me. Believing in yourself is so important. Having people around you who believe in you is also very important to help you through those down days. I'm lucky to have my circle of business-minded Boss Up Babes with me, as well as a little guy who we named Hunter B, who believes in his Mom. I just love him so much; he is the best thing that ever happened to me.

Q: What advice would you give to another boss woman trying to find her way in this difficult time?

Number one, as previously mentioned, is to surround yourself with like-minded people. Surround yourself with solutions-driven people. People who don't use *'shoulda, coulda, woulda,'* or *'can't'*—those are just negating everything you say; it's not worth your time and energy because it doesn't have to be that way. There are so many people out there who are hustling and solutions-driven. We're women; we're moms—we keep going.

In the words of Mama Maria from My Big Fat Greek Wedding, we're the neck that turns the head. In times like these, I think we're the neck and the head. That's what we do. We're women, and we keep going—one foot in front of the other every day. Just surround yourself with people who are like-minded and believe in you.

Then there is self-care. It's so important. Make sure you're getting out, you're doing some exercise, and you're moving. That's so important. And of course, treat yourself once and awhile.

Q: Taking care of yourself. You have your book, Beyond the Banks Success Strategies and Real Estate as a Private Lender. You can definitely check her out. Go to Jodivetterl.com or Beyond the Banks Academy. You're doing a project with your son. You were just telling me about it before the call, Kidpreneur Project. Tell me a little bit about that before we go.

I'm so excited because one of the things I always thought if I ever had a child, I would do a kidpreneur. I was a kidpreneur, even though, that term wasn't a thing back in the 70s and early 80s—to the best of my knowledge. I am very inspired, and I started working with this family, who call themselves The Unstoppable Family—Rhonda and Brian Swan. They have a daughter named Hanalei, and she is so extraordinary. She's the ultimate kidpreneur. She is 12 years old and had her own fashion line. She was the keynote speaker at Burning Man in 2019. She's written a book and developed a kidpreneur program. She uses only sustainable products. She's an ocean ambassador, on and on—she's phenomenal and inspiring.

They live in Bali, and they are American. She has a studio with nine employees, and she runs it. Hanalei designs the product, manages her staff, deals with all the numbers, and gives to charity. Her employees who sew for her were let go when COVID-19 first hit. Then she thought, *you know what, what if I designed face masks?* And so she hit the drawing board, did some prototyping and created these awesome masks from bamboo, so they're soft and comfy on the face. They sent a sample of the masks to Johns Hopkins in Chicago for testing. They tested between 92% and 97% effective for stopping the droplets if you cough or sneeze in the mask or if somebody coughs or sneezes at you. They created a new revenue stream with an employment opportunity for over 100 Balinese to sew and wholesale these masks.

I thought, *why not do this for our first kidpreneur project? It's* been fun and educational for Hunter to launch a little business program with him. He delivers the masks locally by wagon, scooter, or bike, and we are looking forward to dropping off a check at the Food Bank as we have been saving proceeds from each mask sale so Hunter can learn to give back as part of his business. More and more people rely on food banks with the pandemic, so it's a valuable time to give to Food Bank organizations.

Q: I love that idea. Jodi, I look forward to also doing a lot of collaboration soon. Thank you so much.

Thanks so much for having me, Tam. I love getting to know you and talking to you on this podcast. It's fantastic. Love what you're doing.

"Always

believe

in yourself"

—KAREN MEADE

CHAPTER 14:

"Implementing unforgettable customer experiences"

with Yamilca Rodriquez

I AM SO excited today to be talking to my next guest. She is an amazing entrepreneur and activist that I met recently while looking for women who are bossing up.

Q: First of all, welcome Yamilca.
Thank you. I'm so excited to be here.

Q: I'm so excited to have you. So, first of all, where are you calling from?

I'm actually calling from Louisville, Kentucky.

Q: Yes, Louisville, Kentucky. I remember going down to Louisville a lot. We had a lot of family friends from there because our family is from Cincinnati, Ohio.

Right, and I lived in Cincinnati for 20 years.

Q: But I also hear a little bit of an accent. Where are you originally from?

I'm originally from Caracas, Venezuela.

Q: So what got you from Caracas to Louisville and Cincinnati?

Well, that's a long story. I was born in Caracas and then my father did his PhD in California, so we lived in California for six years. That was amazing. I love California, so I'm a little jealous of you right now. And then we went back to Venezuela, and then my dad was offered a job in Macomb, Illinois, middle of nowhere. So we lived there for a year and then we went back to Venezuela and stayed there. We were in the mountains, not in Caracas anymore, but we lived in the Andes mountains for a long time. My parents still live there. And then I decided to come to Cincinnati to attend university. I studied industrial design at the University of Cincinnati.

Q: That's a very good school, by the way. I went there for a year.

Yes, it was number one in industrial design school in

the country, so it's a very, very good school. I worked at Procter and Gamble for 13 years. And then, I moved to Louisville, Kentucky, because I found my sweetheart.

Q: Because of a boy, of course.
Because of a boy, yes. He's actually Br. He's not from Louisville, but he's lived here for a long, long time. Just about as long as I had lived in Cincinnati. So we're both foreign, I guess, foreign born, but we love Louisville. I've been here five years and I just love it. It's a very quaint, small city—a lot smaller than Cincinnati, obviously—but it's very sweet, lots of great food, lots of bourbon. And people like bourbon!

Q: Oh, yes, for sure, Kentucky bourbon, of course.
So, yeah, it's a great city. We live in the middle of nowhere, so it's nice; nobody's around.

Q: Yes. I love that part of the country. So you went to the University of Cincinnati where you got your B.S. in industrial design and your MBA. Then you went on to collaborate with some of the best graphic design and advertising agencies in the nation and design comprehensive brand strategies and consumer product innovations. I think, when we got connected, someone said I should meet you because we both had a background in marketing. You also facilitated more than 70 design thinking sessions around the world, which is amazing.
I did.

Q: And you were crafting brand visions and stories. And I know that you also began doing something called the archetype method for companies to gain more in-depth understanding of the customer. This is where I think a lot of people need help because they have these businesses, but they don't know who they're trying to get. We all talk about customer avatars, we talk about target markets, and you're really digging into who that person is and understanding that, which I think is very important. But you haven't always done that, so what got you there? What got you interested in design and branding and marketing? What was it that you did before?

When I was six years old, I loved drawing; it was my favorite thing. I also loved people, right, I love working with people, talking to people. I didn't ever want to be alone. I have two brothers and three sisters and my parents, a big family, so I was always with people. And so, over time I started to build empathy for others, I guess that's what I would call it. And I had the opportunity to work at Procter and Gamble and we did a lot of research. We went all over the world, talking to people, meeting people in their homes, which is really rare. You don't usually get to visit somebody's home when you're in China. So it was really, really great for me to see that.

But let me go back a little bit and say that when I was figuring out what I wanted to be, like what career path I wanted to take, I remember I was going to be an engineer. Luckily, my dad's friend was at the house one day, and he was talking to me and he was like, "You do not want to be an engineer". I'll tell you, I'm an engineer;

that is not the career for you." He asked, "What do you like to do?" And I said, "Well, I like to draw, but what can I do with that? You know, there's nothing I can do in school with drawing." And he was like, "Oh, yes, there is. There's a graphic design program."

And so I started in graphic design and from there I switched to industrial design. I actually started industrial design in Venezuela and then moved to Cincinnati and finished my program there. We had Procter and Gamble right there, that's where the headquarters are. So I started in innovation and did a lot of innovation work at Procter and Gamble. I moved to brand identity where I got to work with these amazing, globally known agencies. I got to work around the world and facilitated a lot of sessions. I learned a lot of different programs. They had the budgets, they had the resources, and I met who is now my business partner today.

She worked for one of those agencies and we did a lot of work together. She was an expert in archetypes. And so that's where my passion for archetypes came from. It became our foundation for everything we did. We worked together for 10 years straight. Every project we took on, we would map it out. What was the archetype? What was the strategy? What did we need to do to get there? What were our products? What was the innovation? And so, it just kind of came naturally to me, and I did a lot of persona work too, creating personas for people. This love for understanding people and culture really drove me to the archetype method. And what we discussed a little bit before it was the beginning of our journey into the archetype method. A lot of people have a hard time with their superfan, or what they call the strategic target or avatar, whatever you want to call it.

And we discovered that if we can map your primary archetype, we can map your superfan. So it's the psychological approach instead of trying to figure out on your own, because that's really, really hard. This method naturally attracts your Superfan. We have done over a 1000 case studies over the last 10 years and recently as well and it's so fascinating to me how everything fits this perspective psychologically.

Q: Isn't that interesting? So, obviously, as a business strategist and business coach, I'm working with people on their avatar. For me, I think my personal avatar is me 10 years ago, right? I'm just taking a person down the same exact path that I already know works. Does that have a lot to do with it or is it way deeper than that?

So, basically, with archetypes, you can do it through your personality. Because people don't understand branding at all.

Q: At all. It's so funny you said that because I was just talking to someone else who was in marketing. I said, "You know, a lot of marketing people don't really even understand branding."

That is so right. No, they don't. They have no idea. And I was in a company that was all about brands, right? We worked on billion-dollar brands. I was not allowed to work on million-dollar brands. I was only allowed to work on brands worth billions.

Q: Can I stop you for a second? I want this to be clear to people. Yamilca worked on billion-dollar brands. That means people were spending a lot of money to figure out who their perfect person was. And they drill down and research while a lot of small businesses, don't give it a second thought. We're just throwing something out there without considering it. It makes me crazy.

Yes, they make me crazy too. You can't force people to develop their brands. But I wanted them to have an easy, understandable process they could see themselves in and say, "Oh, this makes sense," and have the language to then communicate it. Because let's say you're a business owner and you have a brand and you're working with somebody to build some pages for you. You have the vocabulary to communicate what they're not doing right, or what you want. So what has been amazing about this process is that people now have the knowledge and power to talk to somebody else about their brand in a clear and effective way.

The second thing is that psychologically you naturally attract your Superfan, what we call the opposite and this magnetic attraction to the opposite archetype. We developed this entire process around opposites. I don't think you'll find that anywhere else. But basically when you select your primary brand archetype, you have an archetype that is attracted to your primary archetype which is your opposite. We've built this entire method around the ascension model. Let's say you're a ruler, then your opposite is a magician. So let's study the magician to attract them. By using words they like. This is the messaging you have to communicate.

So now you have your superfan and you can create a lot of messaging and language around that superfan so they will be attracted to you. And you're not reaching them at a superficial level; you're really reaching them on a deep, emotional level.

Q: Right, because there are psychographics, you really have to understand what motivates them.
Yes, so you speak their language, you explain things from their perspective, you put pictures that they are attracted to, and they'll be like, whoa, this is my person.

Q: Right, deeply connecting with people instead of fumbling around and maybe making a connection.
Making things generic, that's not helpful. I teach a lot of design thinking as well, and that's just problem solving, creative problem solving. And I always tell people you can't be general; you have to be specific. What's the problem you're trying to solve? What are the needs and pain points you're trying to deliver or accomplish?

Q: Yamilca, every single business needs to be working with you or getting clear on this, especially if they're serious. Because you can keep fumbling around for a while, but that's going to be the main difference, I think, to really nailing it.
You're right. When you're at the cusp of going from one zero to the next zero, you have to transform. And to be able to transform, you've got to understand what you're going for. And what we say is brand clarity, brand certainty, and that's what it gives you.

Q: Yes, yes. And that's what you call a serious bossing up, right?

Serious bossing up.

Q: Serious bossing up, because you can't really do the same thing you are doing to get the six figures and get the seven; it's a different thing.

You can't.

Q: It's interesting. So what do you think is your biggest hurdle that you've had to overcome to start your own business?

A lot of hurdles. I actually started with a whole different business at the beginning because I have this passion for fashion, I guess. And I was a fashion producer for about two years and realized that it wasn't really giving me what I needed. It was giving me the creative piece, but it wasn't giving me the intellectual drive. You know, what I was doing for so many years that I so thrived on, and the knowledge I held that I wanted to give to other people. And so, I actually made that switch last year. Understanding where to put your energy is really, really hard. Because I thought that people were asking me to keep my fashion business going, and it was so hard to break away from it because people wanted me to keep doing fashion, but it wasn't serving me.

And that was a really hard decision for me, to switch and really focus on this branding piece that I want to take to the world. I started last year with creating courses. But this January was when I figured out this piece, the superfan, and how important it is for people. I mean, I've done this forever, but I just didn't realize how critical it was for businesses to really understand that. So now I'm taking it in that direction, and I'm fully moving forward with it. I've created this archetype quiz, so I'm super excited about that.

Q: Yes, I think it's a good move, You have 25 years of experience or more working with branding and client identity and superfan stuff. That is what you've been doing for billion-dollar companies—billion with a B.

Yes, but sometimes it's so funny how we get stuck in these things, right? When, I started, I was trying to bring it together, but something got my attention and I kind of went in another direction. But I'm back. I'm back on track and I'm really, really excited about expanding this and bringing it to everybody who really needs it.

Q: It's all part of the journey because a lot of people feel bad for doing one thing then making a switch. That is no problem because that's a part of the learning process.

It is. You have to go through the threshold to come out transformed. And, actually, it was interesting even this year because I had been working on this kind of on my own. Although my business partner and I had worked on it together, she had to go in a different direction. But we came back together in January and I'm super excited to have her on board because the both of us can just take on the world.

Q: What is something you have personally faced in your life—your obstacle, your challenge—that you have had to work through?

So, one of the challenges I've had to work through is actually trusting. Trusting myself, trusting my intuition, trusting that what comes up for me is something I should be moving forward with. And that's been really, really challenging. And we talk about mindset. You know, a lot of people talk about mindset and it's not fluff; it's real. If we don't have the right mindset, we will not move forward. People always ask me, "You say you're going to do something and you do it. How does that happen for you?" I say, "It doesn't happen to me. I decide to do this and I will do it, no matter what." That's just the way I am. And I think that's my strength, right? Not everybody has that strength. You know, I sometimes think I'm not doing the right thing. I question what I do all the time. But then, something good happens and I move forward. And then something bad happens and maybe I take three steps back, but then something else happens. it's just part of the journey, I guess.

Q: It's part of the journey, but that's really good. I think a lot of people have to work on their personal trust. How do you stay motivated? What do you do that keeps you in the zone, focused and believing in yourself?

That is key. With all that's happened in the last few months, what I've learned is structure. Structure gives you freedom. Structure, structure, structure. So I wake up, and I meditate. Meditation has really given me that calmness and direction. And meditating is not like thinking through these problems. It's actually not thinking, right, kind of making your brain blank. And so it's really been good for me. That's really helped me in this process. The other thing I do is I exercise. I have time, I'm not commuting, especially you in Los Angeles, but you're not commuting, so why don't you take that time and exercise? I've been really focused on exercising because that gives me energy. And then after I exercise, I study, because I want to educate myself on a new thing or a new process. And then I make all my calls after that and work. I'm working a lot these days because there are a lot of things I want to do, a lot of things I want to bring out. I'm working on different things. It's the same project, but it's case studies and podcasts and reports and all these other things I want to do in the world. Now I actually have the time to work on those things.

Q: Yeah, very good. What advice would you give to an entrepreneur who's sitting here now and thinking, You know, this was tough. I don't know what to do. I don't know if I'm going to be successful. Oh, I just started my business, and now what? What would you tell them to do?

You know, I asked myself those questions as well. And what I would say is there are different ways to get inspired. Like, I sometimes just go outside in nature and get inspired. I would say, try something different. I forgot how that saying goes: if we always do the same thing, we get the same result. So what I would say is, try something different. Try something you haven't tried before, be patient with yourself, and do some self-care, especially women. I mean, a lot of times we just hustle and work and we forget about taking care of us. You know, having those five minutes to ourselves. And so what I would say is, go inward, try to go inward, try to see what your needs are inside and satisfy those, and then take that outward.

Q: Yeah. I think those are great tips. Yamilca, it's been such a pleasure talking to you and I love what you're doing. Definitely check her out at archetypemethod. com. I think she even has a free quiz on there.
I do. Actually, I forgot to tell you, I switched my quiz to brandarchetype.co.

Q: Oh, brandarchetype.co, perfect.
Yes, so get the quiz, the free quiz on brandarchetype.co.

Q: Okay, I love it. This is so good. I'm glad we're going to be planning together for a little while. I definitely see it as collaborating for a long time, because what you do I don't do, but I think it's super necessary. I'm loving that we're getting to know each other more and thank you so much for doing this.
Oh, thank you, and I'm really excited to get to know you more and work with you some more. I'm very excited about this book!. Thank you, Tam, for everything.

CHAPTER 15:

"Mompreneurs; Find Your Focus"
with Clara Capano

═══════════════════════════════════════

ALL RIGHT, SUPERWOMEN. I am really excited to have my next guest. She is the owner of Capano Consulting and spent 15 years supporting working women and mompreneurs, an international trainer, a business coach with Ninja selling systems, as well as the author of *Find Your Focus: 52 Weeks of Clara-ty.*

> **Q: Clara Capano, how are you?**
> I'm fantastic. Thanks so much for having me here.

Q: Yes, I'm so excited, and where do you live?

My primary residence is in Denver, Colorado.

Q: You have been working in coaching women for a while. What actually got you started doing that?

Well, I fell into it by accident. When I was young, I had this passion. I remember telling people that my ultimate goal was to work with individuals and help them learn better communication skills. Given that I was young, everyone didn't believe that it existed. At this stage of my life, I now know that my passion and goal as a young girl was called industrial psychology. On my path to greatness, I decided I needed to enter the field of law. I wanted to be a judge. On my way to law school, I realized that wasn't the path for me. Then, I was introduced to this amazing woman in real estate. She ran a high-performance team, and she was a complete go-getter—very strong, very dynamic, and very charismatic.

I remember after talking with her, I arrived home and told my dad, "I want to be just like her." He said, "Yeah, I kind of knew that would happen." I started working in real estate, and I never had a passion for the actual selling of real estate—but what I loved about it was its fast pace. I loved it as I learned it—because we were on a really big team. We were doing a ton of business, and I was being more of a mentor. I love teaching people how to maneuver through the day-to-day operations. After about six years on the team, I then moved into leadership and that's how I got my first coaching certification. I just knew that's where I was. All this time—growing from the age of about

23 until this point in time—I had my first child, got through a divorce, and I really felt a connection with the working mom because that's who I was.

Even though men are wonderful and there are some great husbands, supporters, significant others out there, the challenges that we face as working moms—running our own business—just are different. I really wanted to create a platform where "that" mom could talk with somebody who knew what she was going through and wasn't going to be just a cheerleader. Someone who can help with some real skills and tools to maneuver all the challenges of running the business, running the household, getting over the guilt and the shame, and all that comes with it. So, they could realize, "You know what, I'm doing okay," and be proud of the role model that they're being for their children while making their mark.

Q: I love this. I saw what it looked like from that space. There are so many things in there as a single mom and entrepreneur. Whether the person they're married to is supportive or not, what is one of the main things you would try to teach married women? That you have to learn to say no, and despite what everyone tells us, you cannot do it all. You can do versions of it, and you can have it all at different stages—but it's not going to be about what we can do because we are capable of doing anything. It's more about what you should do and getting clear on your priorities—knowing that you're going to have to say no and you're going to have to give up certain things—and you've got to be okay with that. I think that's one of the biggest challenges for moms. We have a lot of guilt. We carry the guilt of having a job. We could be telling ourselves or society is telling us, "Why isn't being a mom good enough for you?"

So, we have shame and guilt, and then people still come to us. Again, no matter how wonderful the husband, the boyfriend, the significant other is—I had an amazing ex-husband - But, If the kids get sick, they call mom first. I see it when I'm on the road training. One of the first questions people ask me is, "Who's watching your son?" He's 15 now and much older, but this has been going on for years. We feel like we owe it to so many people and what we end up over-giving to everyone. Then, we are not true and authentic to ourselves. I have learned that being a working mom and running my own company has made me a better mom because I now have my priorities straight. When I am with my son, I am with my son. When I'm with my family, I'm turned off. It has made me much more focused—much more authentic and on purpose with what I'm doing.

Q: Yeah, I love that. You don't have to do everything. If you need to hire or collaborate with someone else, you do it. You don't have to do every single thing.
We need to get over it. For some reason, it's that delegating thing. We have so much guilt and shame around delegating.

Q: We are not getting anywhere with that.
No, because time spent doing one thing is time spent not doing another. I remember I was struggling with hiring a house cleaner. I was feeling guilt and shame, and my mom was the one who reminded me how much I hate doing the job and that hiring someone

gives me extra time with my son or to do something for myself. She's said, "You can make that money that you're paying somebody in one coaching call."

Q: That's right. Let's talk about hurdles. A lot of times, people think we have it all together, which isn't true. What are some of the biggest hurdles you've had to get through?

In no particular order, I think one is to communicate with your support group—whether it's a family member or significant other because they don't always understand it. Especially if you're working with somebody in your world that has a traditional job—the entrepreneur mindset can be very different. I think setting clear expectations about what your goals are, what it is that you're planning to do, what you need from them. It's one of the things I learned in real estate since it can be 24/7, just like any entrepreneurial job. What I found is that telling my family or friends that you have me on Sunday mornings from eight until noon—I'm yours. They will forgive you for the other nights or when you're running behind because when you promise to be there, you are there.

That was one of the things I had to learn. I had to set clear expectations of what I needed from them so that they understood. A big part of my job is being on the road, and I remember having a conversation about it because my son was much younger. I'm on the road probably a good 30–35 weeks out of the year, and I had to explain that it's not about the money—it's about the impact that I can have. When I started sharing that vision and goals, showing the results, the testimonials from the people and moms that I'm helping, they understood. My ex-husband finally said, "I get it now."

I sit down every year—I've done this for about five years now with Nicholas when I do my business plan—and I share it with him. And I say, "In order for me to get here, this is what it's going to look like. Are you okay with this?" I need to make sure I have his support around it.

That's definitely one of the hurdles, making sure that we're communicating clearly. The other hurdle is getting clear on our "why." It's not always about making more money. My "why" is to become a role model. It's to let other people know that I am only where I am because I have people around me who believed in me when I didn't believe in myself. And helping other women understand it that their vision is rocket fuel, whether it's financial freedom, paying for college tuition, never needing somebody and knowing you can do it on your own. You have to really get connected with that because that's what's going to push you through.

Not every day is great. Not every day is filled with rainbows and unicorns. You got to be able to dig deep on the days that are hard and say, "This is why I am doing it." Another hurdle is burnout. We go and go, so you've got to do self-care. You've got to carve out times for a nothing day or do what you need to do. It's the old adage of when you're on an airplane, "You have to give oxygen to yourself first." It's the same thing. I cannot serve at the level I want to serve. I cannot take care of my clients, my family, my son, and my friends. I cannot be the best version of myself if I'm tired, worn out, resentful—any of those things. You've got to make that a priority.

One of the biggest challenges was learning to balance it all. It is really hard to be a mom, and be present with my son while I am also traveling. I had to learn to ask for help and that is not easy. I had to really share my goals and vision with my x, my parents and friends - i could not do it alone. As my son has grown, he is a huge part of my business planning each year. He knows my passions for helping others and supports me. I also work very hard to make time with him the highest possible quality time, so I am very present when with him.

The other challenge is scheduling. You've got to come up with what your optimal week looks like. You also have to know that you have to adjust. If anything, this time that we're in right now has taught us all about that. Knowing that you can move things, but you only move things in your schedule if it's a health or family issue or if it makes good business sense. We have to start thinking like a CEO and start making decisions at that level.

Q: Give me a real BossUp moment in your life that you had to say, "You know what, this is a challenge, and I have to switch on it."

My boss up moment was when my son was about 4. I was working full time, starting my coaching business, getting my masters and a single mom. I was ready to crack and I kind of did. One night, he came to me when I was working and said, "Mommy you are not paying attention to me". My heart sank. I knew something had to change. I realized in my attempt to "do it all" I was doing nothing great and most of all I was not being there for those that matters most.

For me in that moment bossing you meant being honest and vulnerable. I had to set limits and ask for help. I had to learn to identify the things that were true priorities to me and protect that time. I had to say No so things and also forgive myself for not being "perfect". In doing these things, which certainly took time. I have learned to become a better mom, friend and business woman. I have learned that doing it all is not always the best thing and what we should strive for. I did it and I created it—and I'm very proud of all of those things. A lot of other people said if I can manage all that, they can do it too.

Q: Yeah, that is a big motivator. How do you stay motivated?

I listen and I grow a lot. Growth is huge for me, and I listened to a lot of podcasts. I'm constantly reading and just absorbing information so that I can always become a better version of myself. That's one way to keep myself fresh. I motivate myself by going on vacation. I love being able to see new parts of the world. I go back and work more so I can take another vacation—and that motivates me. I love it when people can say they make more money. Who doesn't like that? But those aren't the things that really feed my soul. What feeds my soul is when my clients tell me, "I was able to go on vacation and be where I needed to be. I was able to pay off my debt. I was able to accomplish these things that I wanted to accomplish." That is what means the most to me because money is money. It's coming back to the important things and allowing them to be present in what they're doing. A lot of those things are what motivates me.

Q: I'm the same way. You got to figure out what your thing is.

My clients really motivate me. I can't show up if I don't do the same thing. I can't tell them to go out and do all of these things if I'm not doing it. Knowing that I'm going to be called out if I don't do it too, when I give them permission to call me out if I'm not doing it, so having that transparency. They know that I'm doing the same exact things, and it's that integrity factor.

Q: Do you have a daily routine?

Absolutely! My morning routine is my secret weapon. I get up at 5:15, and one of the first things I do is have my coffee. If I'm here locally, I will take my dog on a walk and listen to a podcast. If I'm on the road, then I do a workout. I also do written affirmations, I do a gratitude practice, and then at least two handwritten notes to somebody so I can work on that. I love doing those.

Q: I got one from you, too. That was so cool.

I look at my schedule and see who I am meeting with. Then, I say, "What are the big three things I need to accomplish today?" I don't want to overwhelm myself with a to-do list of 10 or 15 things. Sometimes, it's okay—I've got to make these calls, I've got to work on this report, I've got to write this article. Sometimes, I've got to go to the post office and buy stamps. I've got to go to the store and buy dog food, but then I can piece it together and say, "I'm picking up Nicholas at school, so I can go to the grocery store before that," so I can then identify those items.

Then, I jump into my emails, voicemails, and go about my day. I also have an end-of-the-day routine. I truly believe in gratitude and what you focus on. So, I start and end my day with gratitude. At the end of the day, I focus on three great things that happened within the day. I think as we get so busy, we tend to focus on all the things we don't get done. Then we start spiraling.

Q: That's awesome. What advice would you give to a mom for things they should do and be more motivated to start a business?
One thing is to do it. Don't feed into the fear. I don't live with regrets, but if I did have one, it would be that I should have done it sooner. I was fearful of all the things that we get fearful of. I would say, "If this is something you really want to do, do it. Don't put a timeline on it." The direction you go is so much more important than the speed at which you go. The second thing is to get a support group. Make sure that you have people because it is hard. You need to make sure that you have some people that you can go to.

You're going to have some mentors. Some that are going to be cheerleaders and some that can help you with strategies, but you've got to work on that and really surround yourself with inspirational people. Then, be honest about your time. You're going to be excited, and you're going to want to jump into it. There are going to be some days when you can work eight hours, and there will be days when you can work for 15 minutes. Set your week up for success, and do the best you can. At the end of the day, you did give the best you could. That's 15 minutes—excellent—just really be honest about the time that you have to invest, and use that time to its highest and best use.

Q: That's great. You have another book coming out aside from an amazing collaboration in Women Who BossUp.

Yeah, I do. I'm working on my second book. We're still working on the title, but it's going to be a guidebook all about unleashing the mompreneur. It's not just going to be some antidotes and just some 30,000-foot views. It's going to be some specific tools for building your vision, creating habits, communicating, and taking care of yourself. We're working on that, and hopefully, it's going to be out in the spring. In the meantime, I'm working on a lot of articles and collaborating with you. Then, I'm also creating a coaching program for the mompreneur. That is a precursor to the book and start working with some people. I'm going to do a small little focus group, and then launch that, hopefully, in a couple of months.

Q: Yes, I love this. Where do we find you?

On Instagram under the Entrepreneurial Mom. On Facebook, they can find me at Clara Capano or Capano Consulting. I am also on LinkedIn—just Clara Capano. On Twitter, I use @clara-ty. Then, my personal website is www.clara-ty.com. I also have a YouTube channel called Moments of Clara-ty.

Q: Can you talk about Moments of Clara-ty?
Every Friday I do a little video blog with just one-minute moments of clarity.

Q: Thanks so much, Claire, for playing in the sandbox with me.
Thank you, I loved it.

LET'S START THERE:

Who do you have to become?
with Tam Luc

═══════════════════════════════════

THE ENTREPRENEUR'S JOURNEY is a journey of personal development. It is the pursuit of becoming better, uplifted, and elevated as well as working on your mindset. There was a quote that always resonated with me. "It's not about the destination, it's who you have to become to get to the destination." In order to believe that you have to know that it's possible. Logically, we know that if one human being can get to a destination, then it's possible for other human beings to do so. What is the difference? Mindset. We keep working on that mindset so that we can become the type of person that would actually get there. Despite the distractions, interruptions and commotions.

One of my client's core beliefs was life is hard for her. She grew up in a hard situation. Her parent's life was hard. Growing up was hard. Even into her forties life was still very hard. I noticed that she was a fighter. But what would it be like if she decided that life wasn't hard? What if she'd believed life was easy and she brought forth easy to her. What if it was possible to attract easy into her life? That would require a mindset shift. Who would she need to become to have it easy? Who would you need to become to be successful? That is the journey of an entrepreneur. It is very much personal development driven, and you can't do one without the other. So today, start with that.

"Whatever you are
going through,
Remember:
You are a Diamond!"

—TAM LUC

What is your story?

What was your epiphany?

When was your Bossup moment?

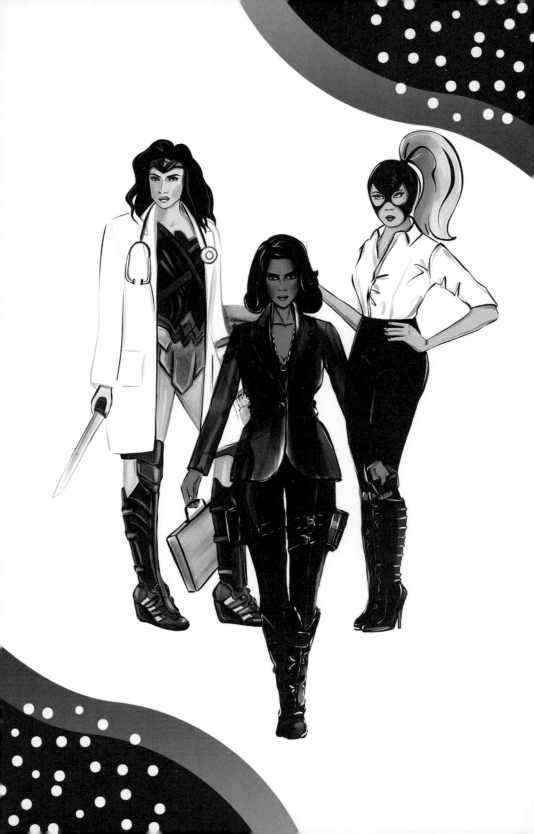

RESOURCES:

Contributors' Biographies

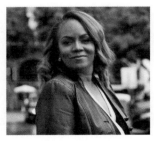

TAM LUC
tam@delucslife.com
www.delucslife.com

Ta Luc has been an entrepreneur and investor since 2002. Being raised by two successful entrepreneurs, she always desired to create the exact same lifestyle as her parents. But instead: she struggled.

For 17 years as a side-hustling entrepreneur, "Stuck like Chuck," Tam Luc was in a job she hated. She had no time for all the things that were important to her until she figured out why. She asked herself the question. "What the hell are you here to say?" She found her answer and discovered that her super-power gift is to help empower women to be seen and heard with brand message strategies.

She's now a No. 1 best-selling author, speaker, blogger and coach who focuses on helping entrepreneurs monetize their message and create a lifestyle that gives them joy.

Tam Luc is the Amazon best-selling author of numerous books, including: "A Woman's Side Hustle," "There's Somebody In My Room," and "The Right End Of The Chase."

"Let's get clear on your message and use it as a tool to create products, customers, sales, and strategic partnerships, advertising, and content," said Tam Luc. "If you are ready to clarify your message and monetize it, enjoy more credibility, and stand out from the crowd then we can definitely help you."

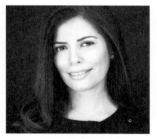

YAMILCA RODRIGUEZ

contact@yamilca.com

www.brandarchetype.co

Yamilca Rodriguez is an artist, entrepreneur, and activist, who was born in Caracas, Venezuela. She has collaborated with some of the best graphic and advertising agencies across the nation to design comprehensive brand strategies and consumer product innovations. Aside from that, she has also facilitated more than 70 design thinking sessions around the world, crafting brand visions and stories that span multiple categories and lead highly influential billion-dollar brands.

The Archetype Method helps companies gain a more in-depth understanding of their customers. By defining their brand archetype, they can implement unforgettable customer experiences across multiple channels and touch-points. Envision your future customer's needs, boost customer adoption, and drive the powerful product as well as service demand.

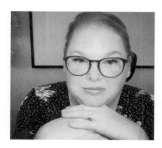

SUMMER HARTMAN

summer@summerssleepsecrets.com

www.summerssleepsecrets.com

Summer Hartman ranked top 200 BEST sleep consultants by tuck.com. She is the Regional Director for the Association of Professional Sleep Consultants (APSC) International Certified Newborn Care Specialist. Aside from that, Summer is also a sleep correspondent for NPR news, Parent.com, and has been seen on AzLiving & regular on Independent talk radio 1100 KFNX.

She is passionate about baby's has created a PROGRAM that has allowed her to teach others. She works with newborns to 6 years old and specializing in sleep training singles, and multiples, also working with reflux and colic. On top of that, she has worked with families in many different capacities through in person, phone, text and VOXER.

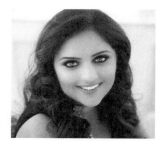

ROMA BAJAJ KOHLI

revive@wellnessbyroma.com

www.wellnessbyroma.com

Roma Bajaj Kohli is a life coach, a host, a motivational speaker, and a leader of a women's empowerment organization. Her global travel adventures and her former experience of being a Global Fashion Apparel Designer has given her the edge to help her clients design and live a life of their best dreams and desires. Her expertise is in helping her clients follow their soul's purpose and passion to become the creator of their own destiny by designing daily practice which helps them be in alignment with their mind, body, and spirit. She currently focuses on key areas such as Self, Work, and Family. She is the founder of 'The Awakened Mind Method ", an 8-week Transformation program that helps soul-centered women leaders master their minds by owning their true power and awakening their innate intelligence through play.

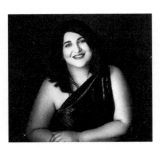

MARISABELLE BONNICI

belle.bonnici@gmail.com
www.roadtobelle.com

Marisabelle Bonnici is the president of the European pharmacy students association between 2008 and 2009. She owned a pharmacy between January 2013 to December 2018. Her biggest struggle was her weight and self-esteem. As a child, she was severely bullied at school as she was always bigger and taller than other girls. She had girls take her to the bathroom and make her throw up so that she would lose weight. As she grew older, this issue kept increasing as she dealt with stress by binge eating. Later on, she sold her pharmacy, worked with a coach who helped her, and now started studying eating disorders and helping others. She is also currently doing coaching courses.

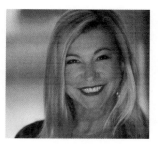

KIMBERLEY LOSKA

aheartspeaks2@gmail.com

aheartspeaks.com

Native to California, Kimberley Loska has motivated audiences, trained leaders, led workshops, and retreats for over 20 years. Kimberley instructs the audience that there is purpose in the pain of life. She is a Keynote Speaker, Certified Life Coach, Speaker's Trainer and serves both men and women through her various coaching programs. Kimberley's goal is to motivate people to change, heal, and freedom. With wholeness and renewal as her goal, she has a passion to exhort and encourage others in their journey towards true transformation. Kimberley knows first-hand how to overcome and survive the trauma and shares her story to let others know that her faith is what got her through her darkest days. She empowers others to Look Up, Reach Out and Step Forward.

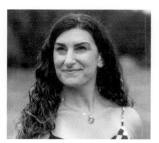

LAUREN D'ANGELO

laurendangelo7@gmail.com

lolayoga.com

Lauren has been active her entire life. Some of her earliest memories are playing outdoors, enjoying nature, and fresh air. In high school, Lauren was an athlete and it was in college when she discovered her love for running. While working in Corporate America, and going to school at night earning her MBA, she hit her first bout of burnout. Soon after, she found her way into a yoga class. Her first class was an experience she said she will never forget, and knew instantly that the practice was something she was supposed to end up sharing. She began regularly practicing in Boston, MA, and was able to manage her anxiety, noticed an overall increased sense of happiness and gratitude, and she was better able to end the space between stimulus and response. Soon after her first class, she set out on a journey to learn to teach and share this practice with as many people as she could. The practice done by yoga goers taught her so much more than physical flexibility. Lauren's goal in creating Lola Yoga is to be a resource. Here you can check my weekly classes and workshops, read her blogs and listen to her podcasts, and even book a private yoga session or corporate event with Lauren. She will share her knowledge of yoga, mindfulness, and health and wellness with you openly.

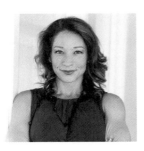

KARISSA WILLIAMS

karissa@365dailyhustle.com

www.365dailyhustle.com

Karissa Williams' coaching practice strives to motivate, educate, and inspire others to live their best lives by offering Signature VIP Coaching Programs and Online Group Programs. Karissa provides clients with the right support, accountability, and fresh perspectives to make lifelong changes when it comes to achieving her client's goals and dreams. As a success coach, Karissa helps stressed-out, career-focused mamas create a better work-life balance. She helps them reset, readjust, and refocus on what's important. Together they build habits that support Self-care, Healthy Living, and Career Growth.

She found her calling as a Coach, Speaker, and Author and brings high levels of energy, motivation, empowerment, and inspiration at any stage. In 2018, she awakened her inner voice. From that space, she reclaimed her authenticity, confidence, and power. Karissa speaks from experience and heart which allows her to BossUp on every level. From sharing her stories with the world, she was allowed to inspire women to rise above and BossUp in life!

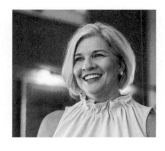

KAREN MEADE

karen@karenmeade.com

www.karenmeade.com

Having worked with hundreds of clients, and with her continued training and research, Karen has a realistic grasp on why people can't always move forward in their home and life. She knows that the act of organizing her client's spaces and their lives is not all that is entailed in her business, but rather it's about building trust, establishing a positive rapport while gently coaching the client, along with celebrating their successes, and providing them with the tools necessary to maintain simple systems. Karen's background is in elementary education, and she has extensive experience in event planning, training, operations, and business management. Living and working in a well-organized, beautifully designed, and aesthetically pleasing space is realistic, no matter the budget. She knows when a client decides they are ready to revamp their home and the life that the fun has just begun.

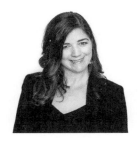

JODI VETTERL

jodi@jodivetterl.com

www.jodivetterl.com

Jodi Vetterl is the author of the book, Beyond the Bank, Success Strategies in Real Estate as a Private Lender. She has a

20-year career in high-tech software sales, and has won multiple sales achievement awards; closed 7-digit deals and enjoyed several President's Club trips around the world. Desiring a career outside of Corporate America, Jodi spent the last 17 years building up a real estate portfolio in both the US & Canada as a passive investor with such strategies as buy & hold single-family homes; investing in multi-family buildings in syndication, and private lending to active investors rehabilitating homes.

As a result of these strategies, Jodi was able to leave Corporate America & establish financial independence at the age of 46 and fulfill her passions around writing, speaking & consulting. She shares private money lending strategies in her book, Beyond the Banks because she enjoys educating others with the resources and knowledge that have helped her create life balance in a more heartfelt way.

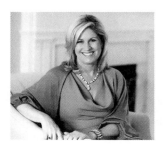

JENNIFER BLAIR

jennifer@excavive.com

www.excavive.com

Jennifer Blair is the founder of Excavive, a life coach, inspirational speaker, entrepreneur consultant, creative motivator, and author. From embracing every moment of motherhood and community involvement to surviving a heartbreaking divorce and reinventing herself with a career she loves today, Jennifer Blair knows how frightening and thrilling change can be. Excavive is a way to empower people to pursue their passions, increase their self confidence, communicate powerfully and build the kind of lives they truly want to live.

Her extensive coaching and leadership skills, as well as personal experiences, allow her to create compassion and trust with her clients to move them forward to envision and embrace their definition of success. Fueled by the desire for intense joy, ignited by her passionate pursuits and motivated by making a positive impact on others, Jennifer strives to live her life with balance, purpose, and passion each and every day, and she inspires her clients around the country to do the same.

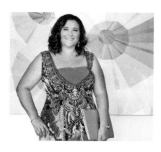

JASMINE KRATZ

jasmine@inspiredimpact.com.au

www.inspiredimpact.com.au

Jasmine Kratz is a mentor for entrepreneurs, small business owners, coaches, and Affiliate and Network Marketers teaching her clients how to create their online empires. Her passion for supporting people and seeing them succeed is what gets her out of bed every day. Her jam is helping you get sexy systems and tailored tools in place to share your brand and your message with the world.

As one of the lead trainers in the Online Entrepreneur community, she teaches online marketing to a community of entrepreneurs. As a business owner, coach, and online marketer she knows exactly how you feel and the challenges that you face in growing your brand online and will support you to get out of the overwhelming phase and start seeing success. Hence why the VIP Branding Days & Empire Growth Retreat was born, a 3-day event to bring together everything you need to dominate your niche and build a successful personal brand online that attracts your ideal clientele.

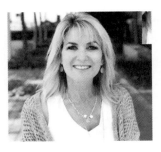

VICTORIA PLEKENPOL

victoria@oylwithoutboundaries.com

www.oylwithoutboundaries.com

Victoria began her international travels in 1994 when she and her husband set off for Hong Kong from her home in California. Over the past 26 years, she has lived in Hong Kong, Singapore, New Jersey, The Netherlands, Edinburgh, Scotland, Shanghai, and now Shenzhen, China. Victoria is now a Sales Executive/Blue Diamond and Founder of dōTERRA China and is working with the company and her team to help open the China Region. With a global team of over 7,000 in more than 50 countries, she has developed an outstanding training and educational system to reach around the world.

She believes the only way people will be able to live fully and fulfill the purpose they were created for is if they are healthy, clear-minded, and full of energy! Her mission is to empower and educate women to OWN their Lives Without Boundaries. To assure them that it is never too late to make a change. To help them discover their purpose and fulfill it.

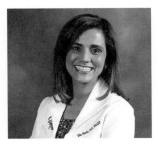

DR. USHA MANTHA

drmantha@yahoo.com

www.vervemedspa.com

Dr. Usha Mantha MD is the founder and CEO of Verve Weight Loss and Laser Aesthetics, a medical spa located in Upland, California in the greater Los Angeles area. Having trained and received membership from the Royal College of

Obstetricians and Gynaecologists in London, U.K., Dr. Mantha has been a Women's Health expert for over 30 years.

She is also a dual Board-Certified physician in Obesity Medicine in California and Family Medicine in Pennsylvania, but she is also a Provider, Instructor, and Advisory Faculty in Advanced Life Support in Obstetrics and Advanced Cardiac Life Support in adults. After decades specializing in women's health, Dr. Mantha trained and became an expert in weight loss management, and has helped hundreds of patients in the Inland Empire with offices in Pomona and Upland, California over the past 15 years. She is Director of Weight and Wellness clinic at Casa Colina Hospital for Rehabilitation, where she treats overweight and obese patients in pre- and post-operative care. She is also a visiting faculty instructor at School of Medicine at Riverside and teaches Family Medicine and PM&R residents at both Casa Colina and Pomona Valley Hospital Centers.

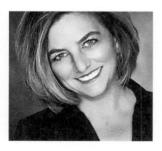

CLARA CAPANO

clara@clara-ty.com

www.clara-ty.com

Clara Capano is the owner of Capano Consulting and has spent over 15 years supporting Working Women and Mompreneurs to grow their business and maintain harmony in their life. She is the author of Find Your Focus: 52 Weeks of Clara-ty, and international trainer and business coach with Ninja Selling Systems.

Native to California, Kimberley Loska has motivated audiences, trained leaders, led workshops, and retreats for over 20 years. Kimberley instructs the audience that there is purpose in the pain of life. She is a Keynote Speaker, Certified Life Coach, Speaker's Trainer and serves both men and women through her various coaching programs.

Kimberley's goal is to motivate people to change, heal, and freedom. With wholeness and renewal as her goal, she has a passion to exhort and encourage others in their journey towards true transformation. Kimberley knows first-hand how to overcome and survive the trauma and shares her story to let others know that her faith is what got her through her darkest days. She empowers others to Look Up, Reach Out and Step Forward.

LET'S BE SOCIAL

Do you have a BossUp moment in your life?
We want to hear your story.
Email us at: support@delucslife.com